D1123636

EVOLVING HEALTH

The Origins of Illness and How the Modern World Is Making Us Sick

Noel T. Boaz

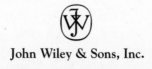

John Wiley & Sons, Inc.

To Homo sapiens,
that they may learn to live with themselves

Copyright © 2002 by Noel T. Boaz. All rights reserved.

Published by John Wiley & Sons, Inc., New York.
Published simultaneously in Canada

This publication is designed to provide accurate and authoritative information in regard to the subject matter covered. It is sold with the understanding that the publisher is not engaged in rendering professional services. If professional advice or other expert assistance is required, the services of a competent professional person should be sought.

Library of Congress Cataloging-in-Publication Data is available from the publisher.

ISBN 0-471-35261-6 (cloth)

Printed in the United States of America

10 9 8 7 6 5 4 3 2 1

Contents

Tables

Acknowledgments

When one embarks on a new journey into vast and intellectually uncharted territory, there are many guides along the way to whom he is beholden. Boyd Eaton, one of the founders of evolutionary medicine, has been a guiding light for many years, and it was he who first crystallized for me the revolutionary idea that paleoanthropology has something to say to medicine. Many colleagues in biological anthropology and medicine have inspired me through discussions and their writings. Frank Johnston, Wayne Calloway, Mike Little, Bill Adams, Barry Hicks, Jim McKenna, Wenda Trevathan, Jack Cronin, Mel Konner, Jack Buchanan, Sean Ervin, Steve Deschner, Barry Hicks, John Patton, Gene Colburn, Agnes LaVille, Gerhard Meisenberg, Gerald Grell, Birgit Nardell, Bill Cain, Alan Almquist, Mustafa Hrnjicevic, Russ Ciochon, Ramesh Krishnamurthy, Paul Simons, and others too numerous to name have all affected my approach and development of ideas. My friends and colleagues associated with the International Institute for Human Evolutionary Research and its foundation—Ken Haines, Paris Pavlakis, Tim Wolf, Boyd Eaton, Mary Smith, Marc Feldesman, Dick Markwood, Bart Queary, Rick Harrington, Bill McCampbell, the late Peter Williamson, and the late Frank Spencer—have my thanks for the myriad ways they helped the project. My editor, Stephen S. Power, has been a long-suffering and insightful critic, and a pleasure to work with. Susan Rabiner, my agent, believed in the book early on. I thank my inspirational children, Lydia, Peter, and Alexander, and, finally, my wife, Meleisa McDonell, M.D., a clinician of the first order, for her patience, support, insight, and endless discussions on the meaning of diseases and how they might have evolved.

At times, I have felt overawed by the immensity of the subject of evolutionary medicine, and concerned that the book would jump tracks from the hypoglossal to the Panglossian, or from the homeotic to the homeostatic. I can only beg the reader's indulgence if I have lingered too long on long-lost organismal details or paid too little attention to certain important topics that should have been dealt with in more depth. I alone am responsible for any misdirected leaps of logic or unwarranted extrapolations that the following pages may contain.

Introduction

It is possible to prevent most modern diseases. Strangely, this secret to health is not waiting to be unveiled by white-coated lab scientists. It has already been unearthed by dusty paleontologists. It is the lifestyle of our ancestors.

Human evolution is the framework for this book, but it is health and prevention of disease that give it its focus. The evolutionary framework is a *scala adaptiva*, made up of evolutionary levels to which each of our adaptations belongs. Our ability to breathe air, for example, is inherited from our amphibian forebears who lived some 300 to 340 million years ago (Level 8 in our scheme, introduced in chapter 2). When something goes wrong with our ability to breathe then, such as in the lung disease emphysema, there is a fundamental unraveling of a Level 8 adaptation that natural selection crafted many, many years ago. By understanding how the adaptation came about and then dissecting how a modern disease deranges that adaptation, we gain a very good idea of the disease. This knowledge helps sufferers of the disease understand and work to alleviate their symptoms, and it helps others prevent the disease.

This book is organized by evolutionary levels. Birth defects and mutations, discussed in chapter 3, are ultimately traceable to failures of adaptations of our extremely remote single-celled ancestors (at Levels 1 and 2). Cases of direct poisoning of our cells, as by mercury, for example, even recall adverse chemical reactions before the advent of life itself (Level 0). Our cells' competition (and coevolution) with viruses is probably almost as ancient, and is discussed in chapter 4. Flu and the common cold are the most familiar modern representatives of Level 2 and 3 diseases. Cancer is a failure of the major adaptation of Level 3, that of cells living together cooperatively, and is treated in chapter 5.

Hormones became important at this same level as ways for cells to communicate, and they mediate such reproductive system cancers as breast carcinoma and prostate cancer, discussed in chapter 6. Heart disease, the number one cause of death in the Western world, originates as a problem of salt and water balance, an adaptation of our fish ancestors at Level 7. It is the topic of chapter 7. We evolved air-breathing lungs as amphibians at Level 8, and failure of this adaptation leads to such diseases as emphysema and lung cancer, dealt with in chapter 8. We developed a perpetual sweet tooth—for the energy-rich sugars and vitamin C in fruits—as early primates in Level 11. Today, carbohydrate-rich sources of sugar lead to diabetes mellitus type II, discussed in chapter 9. Mutations to conserve the body's water occurred at Level 14, in our ape ancestors, the precursory condition for gout (chapter 10). Many musculoskeletal and mechanical problems, such as back pain and flatfeet, track back to our adoption of an upright, two-legged posture as hominids (Level 15 and chapter 11). Chapter 12 discusses diseases of the digestive tract that are failures of our basic hominid dietary adaptation (also Level 15), although some other digestive problems that affect only some groups of people, such as celiac sprue, are of very recent evolutionary origin (Level 17). Psychiatric illnesses (discussed in chapter 13) represent failures of our complex brain—a hallmark of humanity (Level 16). Earlier adaptations then show through, as in obsessive-compulsive disorder, when behavior becomes rigid, stylized, and repetitive, recalling adaptations inherited from our Level 9 reptilian ancestors and controlled by the ancient reptilian parts of our brain.

The second theme in the book is "adaptive normality." By viewing the many levels of human evolution from the present, we can come to understand what our normal ranges of environment, anatomy, physiology, and behavior really are. Our internal body temperature, for example, is normally between 98 degrees Fahrenheit and 99 degrees Fahrenheit, and when it lies outside this, something is wrong. In this book we will seek the evolutionary reasons for why our various gauges are set where they are. We are at thermal equilibrium when the temperature next to our skin is about 70 degrees Fahrenheit, indicating that we humans are at base tropical creatures, evolved over millions of years, mainly on the African continent. Our physiology maintains stability as much as possible around this set point—sweating if we are too hot or shivering if we are too cold. Illness happens when our coping mechanisms with environmental change are overwhelmed or stressed—for example, in fever or hypothermia.

A lack of fit between environmental conditions and the adaptations of an individual is termed "discordance," and it is the major cause of preventable disease in the modern world. If a human being tried to live without clothes, shelter, and fire in the Northern Hemisphere winter, for example, he or she would soon die because of the extreme discordance between our tropical adaptation and the low environmental temperatures. Most of the discordances that we deal with today are of much lower magnitude, but their cumulative effects over time can be no less deadly. Our goal in this book is to reduce discordance and to find the optimal operating ranges or zones for major human adaptations. Seeking adaptive normality is a new concept in medicine, but it is important to you in understanding health and disease, and in maintaining a healthy lifestyle.

Although an integrated evolutionary understanding of health and disease promises a powerful new scientific approach, evolutionary medicine is not yet mainstream; however, it is not "alternative medicine," either. It is firmly grounded in the Western scientific tradition and fully incorporates modern scientific findings. It also has its detractors. James Bull, a molecular biologist at the University of Texas, has called evolutionary medicine "mostly a guessing game about how we think evolution worked in the past—what it designed us for."[1] Of course, like all science, it is guesswork initially, but with the new tools of molecular biology and geochronology, combined with the old methods of comparative anatomy, pathology, and clinical medicine, the hypotheses of evolutionary medicine can be tested. For example, we can decide competing evolutionary explanations of gout discussed in chapter 10 by putting together molecular and paleontological data to date the gene mutations underlying the disease. And we must reassess the paleodietary proscription against eating dairy products (as dietary components too recently evolved to be good for us) because clinical experience has shown that people whose herding ancestors evolved lactase genes in order to effectively digest milk do just fine eating dairy products (chapter 14). Evolutionary medicine is built of hypotheses that can be disproved by scientific data that contradict them or by clinical experience not consistent with predicted outcomes.

Evolutionary medicine promises not only a revolutionary new approach to the science of medicine, but a powerful way for people to integrate a new understanding of health and lifestyle to prevent disease. The most common and debilitating modern diseases can be prevented—by knowledge, and action based on that knowledge. Patients can assume more responsibility for themselves, and as prevention becomes more and more a part of standard medical practice, they can become full partners with their doctors in maintaining their health. By following the suggestions in this book, your quality of life, especially as you age, will stay high, and your life span may actually be lengthened. In medical parlance, the lifestyle changes advocated here will decrease morbidity, likely delaying mortality until older ages than now generally seen. Nothing advocated in the book will hurt you, not even adding insects to your diet (chapter 14), but as you regain your evolutionary birthright and evolve back to health, consult your physician.

1

Achieving Adaptive Normality, Your Evolutionary Birthright

Is it possible that something that makes us feel good might really not be good for us? In nature, animals are adapted to live in a particular way, and they almost certainly derive pleasure from doing the things that they do. Dogs, for example, adapted to hunting in packs, get a kick out of chasing large moving things. In the past these were always elks, moose, wildebeests, and even the odd infirm mammoth. Today, however, if a suburban dog chases down and takes a bite out of the only large prey available to him, the rolling rubber tire of a garbage truck, it could be fatal. What the dog has evolved to like to do is injurious to its health and longevity.

Sometimes even severe object lessons cannot teach the dog otherwise. A dog I had when I was six, Blackie, loved to chase cars. One day Blackie's leg was broken by a mail truck he was pursuing. The vet thought that Blackie should be put to sleep, but we had a cast put on the leg and it eventually healed. I hoped that this painful episode would convince Blackie to reform, but it didn't. Only a few months later Blackie was found smashed in the road and was taken away by the sanitation workers when I was at school. I wondered for years what deep-seated desire it was that made dogs chase moving motor vehicles. After losing two more dogs, otherwise well trained, to similar highway accidents, I eventually concluded that this behavior was hardwired in them—left over from some Pleistocene adaptation that had benefited their species in the past but now was killing them.

Unlike dogs, human beings are omnivorous—scavenging, gathering, and hunting primates who can eat just about anything that crawls, walks, swims, or flies. Although few of us have a problem confusing a car with our next meal, we have a flaw as hardwired as our dogs': fat. Especially tasty to us are food items that are full of fatty acids—energy-rich molecules that become stored around our midsections in fat cells and substances craved by our voracious lipid-rich brains. We also love sugar, a predilection developed by our fruit-eating ancestors who, when they found a tree with ripe, sweet fruit, gorged on it to excess. The realities of our evolutionary past were that fats and sugars were in short supply and famine might hit tomorrow. These evolved tastes were adaptive, and it made evolutionary sense for our hominid ancestors to store up energy reserves for lean times ahead. Today, we store up dessert, eating it even after our stomachs are full, simply because it tastes so good, and building up fat cells that famine will never diminish.

Human evolution is both history and current reality. Its twists and turns have bequeathed to us inborn responses and anatomical traits that serve to adapt us admirably to our many activities and undertakings. But we also obey obviated evolutionary commands. We fear the dark, for example, not because this is a rational decision on our part, but because we are descended from millions of generations of visually oriented, day-living primates systematically preyed upon by nocturnal predators. Amazonian snakes are major predators of New World monkeys still today, and ancient leopards left bite marks on South African australopithecine fossils 3 million years ago. Over the long course of our evolution things that went bump in the night really could kill us. Fear of the dark was an evolutionary outgrowth of natural selection—the more fearful, more vigilant, and thus most quickly reacting individuals avoided being eaten by the snakes, large raptorial birds, and cats that preyed on small-bodied, tree-living primates. Today, innate fear of the dark can still be of survival advantage to us, as when we become nervous and suspicious when walking down a poorly lit urban street at night. But irrational fear of the dark seems to be primarily a characteristic of children, whose small size and experience would have made them most vulnerable to predation in the past. Natural selection hardwired this primate response to danger the same as it did the "freeze-crouch" of a frightened fawn.[1]

Many human traits and behaviors that were adaptive in our evolutionary past may now be maladaptive because the environment in which we arose has changed. In fact, the habitats in which we find ourselves today have changed so drastically and so rapidly from the conditions in which we evolved that it is surprising that we live in them as well as we do. The ultimate irony is that the biggest agent of change in our environment—the architect of our various habitats on Earth—is none other than Homo sapiens.

The Cultural Econiche

Every species has its own econiche—a place in nature where it is at home. An econiche includes not only a physical location on Earth, but the dietary adaptations, daily activity patterns, mating behaviors, and physical attributes that adapt a species to a particular way of life. Hominids, those two-legged creatures that evolved from apes in the African Miocene about 7 million years ago, used to know their place. Their ancestral biological econiche was in the savannas and woodlands of Africa.[2] But their descendants, the human beings, have more recently wandered widely over Earth and have somehow lost this knowledge. As a species, we have lost sight of home.

Culture, the composite of all learned human behavior passed on socially, was the hominids' passport out of Africa and into Eurasia, 1.9 million years ago.[3] Culture makes human beings very adaptable organisms, and it allows humans to cope more rapidly in different circumstances than would be possible left only with their biological rate of evolutionary change. For this reason anthropologists consider that humans have now evolved to live in a new econiche, a cultural econiche.[4] Instead of slowly evolving biologically in response to environmental challenges, humans now evolve bio-logically to bear culture, mainly with their large and complex brains, and culture in turn changes rapidly to adapt to the environment. Humans thus are somewhat unique among animal species in having a cultural econiche within their biological econiche. Traditional Laplander reindeer herders in Finland, for example, have a cultural econiche in the Far North that allows their biological selves underneath to maintain a constant 70 degree Fahrenheit tropical microhabitat inside their warm fur-lined boots and parkas. Nomads in the Negev Desert, on the other hand, wear open-necked, loose-fitting, dark woolen cloaks that shield them from the blistering sun, blowing sand, and cold night-time temperatures. The cloaks absorb heat, creating a vertical cir-culation of air that keeps skin temperature at about 70 degrees Fahrenheit and body temperature normal.

The problem is, culture can adapt us to such a wide variety of conditions that there is a danger that we can diverge so much from our origins that we are in conflict with our biological econiche. Unlike the Laplanders and Negev nomads, whose cultural attri-butes adapt them admirably to their environments, many of our modern-day cultural adaptations may be killing us. We have to adapt culture to suit our biological needs. For example, we know that as early as 2.3 million years ago, our ancestors were wide-ranging, savanna hominids.[5] Today the automobile serves the eco-nomically practical goals of foraging for food and transport back to our home base, but our ancient expenditure of physiological energy for these purposes has been lost. We must figure out how to replace this important biological component of our lives—physical exer-cise—if we want to stay healthy and live long, productive lives. Learning how to shape our cultural behavior to maximize our bio-logical existence is the major goal of this book.

The Pursuit of Adaptive Normality: Average Is Good

Because natural selection has formed them within an ecological niche, species of animals have optimal ranges of structure and function (anatomy and physiology) for all life systems. Most of the individuals within a population will cluster near the mean, average, or norm (used here synonymously) of whatever measure that one looks at. For example, a population of African black-and-white colobus monkeys has an average length of tail, an average coloration pattern, and an average daily metabolic rate. Individual traits of individual colobus monkeys will vary around the mean. No one monkey will be the ideal "type," but still we will have a good idea of a general range of "normal" colobus monkey anatomy and physiology. We humans use this concept all the time when we take a person's temperature, check the health of a growing child by comparing how tall and heavy he or she is against standards for the whole population, or take our own blood pressure. But why are these values normal?

Natural selection tends to maintain an optimal average for a population. Human babies, for example, tend to weigh on average approximately seven pounds. If they are much less or much more than this weight, they have significantly more medical problems associated with their development. The individuals in a population that grow up to be the most successful at survival and reproduction then will tend to have the "average" traits. In a classic study in 1898 on English sparrows that were caught in a snowstorm, ornithologist Herman Bumpus discovered that the birds which survived were nearest the mean in terms of wing length and body size. There were disproportionate numbers of big birds and small birds killed compared to average-sized birds, a gruesome illustration of how natural selection culls individuals too far from the optimum.

Any number of natural disasters befalling a population—drought, floods, freezing temperatures, fire, or, of particular interest to us in this book, disease—may serve as the agents of natural selection. Individuals near the norm for the population tend to survive all of these onslaughts better than the outliers. This type of natural selection is known as "stabilizing selection" because it tends to keep the population on its evolutionary path when overall environmental conditions stay the same. Why exactly it is optimally beneficial for a human baby to weigh seven pounds or for an English sparrow to have a certain wingspan is a hard question to answer. It is probable that "generalists"—individuals not too big but not too slight, not too strong but not too weak—can survive the widest range of hazards. They are not specialized in any one direction and thus tend statistically to survive well. Only if conditions change permanently and in one direction will stabilizing selection be replaced by directional selection, moving the average for the population to a new point.

Biologically speaking, then, average is good and, literally, "normal." Average is, in fact, the best. But extending this concept of evolutionary biology to contemporary philosophy, especially American popular culture, encounters some difficulty. This idea runs counter to many peoples' mind-sets. Asked to predict which birds would survive a storm, most people would probably say either "the strongest birds" or "the biggest birds." Asked to define "best" in human terms, most people would also say "the biggest," "the most beautiful," "the smartest," "the fastest," or "the richest." The *Guinness Book of Records* does not, after all, list *means* of achievement. No one would be interested. So we must first of all separate the ideas of "societal good" from "biological good," for which extremes can mean premature death.

"Good" in a biological sense is "adaptive normality"—a zone in which we function optimally. The unfortunate truth is that many of us operate outside this zone, and we have, by this definition, abnormal lifestyles. Abnormal lifestyles predispose us to chronic illness and "diseases of civilization." Instead, we need to be closer to the biological averages that are at the center of our adaptation as a species.

To achieve adaptive normality, then, should we emulate Neandertals, early hominids, and our ape relatives? In certain important respects, yes. But this does not mean donning a leopard skin and swinging through the trees. Adaptive normality does not imply a reversion to prehistoric cultural conditions, just a simulation of the essentially important conditions within which we evolved.

Our occupations and professions are specialized jobs within culture that deprive us of much of our evolutionary birthright. We do a small number of tasks over and over, and we become very good at them. But despite our competence we become bored with our jobs. We have evolved a complex brain, with matching physiology and anatomy, to deal with a kaleidoscope of changing conditions—threats to our survival—and the mundane sameness of our everyday modern lives creates a chronic discontent. Our psychology tells us that something is wrong, but our intellect fails to analyze how to correct it. We are, in fact, operating at one of the edges of our adaptive zone—in one small place where chance, economic forces, our own interests, and culture have placed us. If we stay there, eventually our health deteriorates. Our cultural econiche adaptation is significantly off the biological norm, and, like a bird that is too big or too small, we will likely die early.

Take Sonya Haskins,[6] for example. Sonya works in a chicken processing plant in Georgia. Sonya's job is cutting off the feet of the chickens as they come down the conveyor belt, in one deft swift motion, putting the feet in one bin and replacing the now footless chickens on the belt. She works eight hours a day—ten sometimes, if she can do the overtime. She hates the work, but she has to support her two small sons. Her back, shoulders, and feet always ache after a day of this work, but she considered herself young and strong when she started and has kept at it. After six years on the job, however, Sonya's hands began to go numb and moving them became painful. She was diagnosed with bilateral carpal tunnel syndrome, underwent surgery on both wrists, and is now recuperating. Her doctor advises her to find another line of work after she gets off disability. Probably not bad advice, but Sonya's physical problem was brought on by an abnormal work environment, and anyone subjected to similar stresses would have the same ailments. What about the thousands of other Sonyas out there in similar situations? Sonya is just being asked to move from one abnormal margin of her adaptive zone to another edge—a sort of slash-and-burn approach to life and health in the modern world. Should Sonya have other options? Yes. Will she get other options? The unfortunate answer is probably no, unless she takes a longer view and moves herself to a more normal and well-balanced position in her work and life. This is what this book is about: understanding adaptive normality and how it came about, and then using that information as a life strategy.

Benton Hawthorne is a 45-year-old corporate vice president in a large city. His job is to analyze sales figures, assess performance of employees, and attend meetings. His job creates a lot of stress—people he has to confront, and even fire, trying to push others to meet goals that never get met, and keeping his superiors happy. Benton was athletic in school, but his hectic lifestyle, plus commuting two hours each day (if the traffic is not too bad), has prevented him from getting the exercise that he knows he needs. Somehow there's never time. He rarely eats breakfast, grabbing a quick coffee and doughnuts, and frequently skips lunch. Yet he is dissatisfied with his weight and his appearance, and now his stomach has begun to act up. He's afraid he has an ulcer, and the pain is beginning to keep him up at night. He hasn't told anybody, not even his wife, but he also is having problems with hemorrhoids, which make sitting through seemingly interminable meetings even more painful.

Benton is working on developing a number of modern-day medical problems simultaneously. His lack of exercise is contributing to his weight gain, and he is at risk for developing diabetes. His diet and his stressful lifestyle are contributing to his stomach pain, which is likely gastritis, preliminary to peptic ulcer. His sedentary routine is also causing a pooling of blood in the walls of his recto-anal canal, causing hemorrhoids. He can expect even more problems, such as back pain, heart disease, kidney disease, and a variety of possible cancers, unless he reverses course and changes his behavior.

Benton is on the opposite end of the economic scale from Sonya, but he is in the same boat from the standpoint of his health. It is deteriorating because of lifestyle choices. Neither Sonya nor Benton really need a doctor to tell them that what they themselves are doing is causing their maladies, that their diseases are preventable, and that their behavior patterns are changeable. The medicine they need is prescribed by our evolutionary history, and it is called adaptive normality.

Concordance and Discordance

Choosing extremes leads to a lifestyle that is "discordant" with our biological evolution. By contrast, "concordant" behaviors are those that play the same adaptive role for us in our present-day environments as they did for our hominid ancestors in their ancient environments. Concordant behaviors bring our biological econiche closer to our cultural econiche. For example, when we walk into our kitchen to make the morning coffee and step, barefoot, on a sharp piece of glass left over from a child's accident the night before, our foot immediately recoils, preventing penetration of the sharp object into our foot. This behavior is identical in context and adaptive value to an *Australopithecus afarensis* pulling back his or her foot when accidentally treading on an upturned acacia thorn, left over from a giraffe's breakfast, while walking along the savanna at Laetoli, Tanzania, 3.6 million years ago. This foot recoil behavior is thus concordant behavior—same environmental problem, same physiological response, same physical effect.

Now let us look at some discordant behavior. After avoiding the painful acacia thorn, our australopithecine walks on a ways and starts to get hungry. He happens to see a Pliocene giant East African tortoise (now extinct) plodding through the undergrowth, and he begins to think how good the fat on the tortoise's back under the shell, the succulent organs, and the salty blood will taste. He gives chase as it were to the tortoise, kills it with a rock, and spends an hour smashing and prying open the carapace. He and his band spend the rest of the day eating the tortoise and resting in the shade. It will be a good many days or weeks before the band will again have this much good food all at once. In contrast, back in the modern world and having forgotten our early morning incident with the broken glass, we find ourselves later in the day, shopping with our seven-year-old son. He begins roaming the supermarket aisles, scanning for game. He happens to see an entire row of potato chips, and he begins to think how good these fat-soaked, salty, fried sliced tubers would taste. Acting on his ancient cravings for these tastes, he lunges and captures a bag of them. But feeding on this low-fiber, high-fat, and high-sodium junk food, coupled with the fact that almost no calories were expended in obtaining them, contributes to obesity, arterial plaque formation and high blood pressure, and diverticular disease of the colon. Our modern behavior in this case is thus discordant with our evolutionary past.

Evolutionary medicine does not advocate returning to the past. Modern medicine has indeed made major strides in overcoming infectious disease, treating trauma, and significantly reducing infant mortality. But if we moderns can consolidate these advances and live in accordance with the evolved wisdom of our bodies, we will achieve optimal health.

Conquering the Diseases of Civilization

The stunning accomplishment of sequencing the human genome, accomplished during the year 2000, is the capstone of an impressive array of discoveries in medically relevant genetics and molecular biology during the latter half of the 20th century. But as impressive as these strides have been, they will not resolve the scourge of modern medicine—the so-called diseases of civilization:[7] heart disease, most cancers, diabetes, and obesity.

How do we defeat diseases of civilization? These are diseases caused not by single gene defects but by the crowded, stressful, polluted, and "modern" conditions in which we human beings have surrounded ourselves in the last several millennia. The diseases of civilization will not be conquered primarily by medical advances in the genetics and molecular biology laboratories. Rather, the diseases that are killing and debilitating most Americans today are lifestyle diseases—discordances with our evolved adaptations that must be reversed by old-fashioned behavioral modification.

As medical genetic research moves rapidly forward, the genetic bases of our adaptations will one day become more fully understood. Hopefully, this understanding will help to teach us how genes function when we are healthy, rather than only how they cause disease. This ability to define the normal—that is, how our bodies and physiologies are designed to function in a disease-free state—is perhaps the major contribution that an evolutionary approach can give to medicine. Genetics should be an active partner with an evolutionary perspective in this endeavor. Throughout the remaining chapters in this book, genetics forms an important part of the evolutionary narrative. The next chapter outlines the broad scope of human evolution, providing a 17-level framework for defining human adaptive normality.

2

How Our
Health Evolved

Doctors focus on disease—how it comes about, how to prevent it, and how to get rid of it. But we, as preventicists, are concerned with health—medically defined as "the absence of disease." We would like to prevent disease because it may be difficult to get rid of, its effects may be long lasting, and, of course, you do not feel very well while you have it.

Health is more than simply the opposite of sickness. From a physiological standpoint, health is optimal functioning of all body systems. This definition is a bit difficult to put into practice because the only way to experimentally determine optimal functioning of an organ or a system is to examine it in isolation—not really what we want to know. What we need to get at is the proper range of activity for an organ within a normally functioning human body. We need to look at the entire organism for this.

As soon as we begin to look at the entire human organism we are confronted with complexity—mystifying complexity. One part interacts with another part; a hormone from one tissue of the body affects another tissue; an invading microorganism prompts a defensive response that then causes a cascade of physiological effects; different external circumstances change the internal environments of our bodies; exogenous chemicals or infecting viruses may damage our genes; food and water are being ingested; waste is being eliminated. Sometimes all of this may be happening at the same time. So far, no one has invented a biological monitoring system sensitive enough and a computer program powerful enough to keep track of all the potentially important physiological states that we may be experiencing at any one moment and to which we may be switching within the next second or two. A rigorous physiological definition of health is thus elusive. Physiologists do the best they can to express the ideal, cooperative interaction of all the body's system by invoking the single term "homeostasis," which means "maintaining sameness" within the body. They speak of the "wisdom of the body."

Lacking a rigorous physiological definition of health, doctors fall back on trial and error. For example, if one kidney fails, doctors know that the body can survive on the other kidney, if it is healthy. The second kidney takes up the slack and homeostasis is maintained. Doctors can say in this case "your kidney is healthy," but they are generally more cautious in issuing a patient a clean bill of health. They know too well that a body struggling to maintain homeostasis is hardly optimal. When stress is put on one system, other interacting systems may be affected. The system under stress will also likely wear out or fail sooner. The doctor then has to intervene. In this case, he or she might prescribe dialysis to remove the body's toxic wastes that are no longer taken out by the kidneys. So what we need is a definition of health that is in agreement with traditional medical and physiological definitions, but also one that gives us some positive guidelines. When are we in good health? When are we in bad health? How can we analyze this state and do something about it?

Good health is physiological homeostasis at all levels of our physical makeup—molecular, cellular, tissue, organ, and organismal. These levels of organization evolved, and the original adaptations were self-contained and independently functioning. Now all levels are subsumed within and mutually integrated into a normally functioning human body. We are, in a sense, a Russian doll, which is composed of successively smaller—that is, earlier

evolved—dolls, eventually shrinking down to the size of a molecule. Each doll was, and still is to a certain extent, a system unto
itself, even though evolution has crafted interdependence of the
systems through time. Because evolution has built us this way, it
makes biological sense to define health as the normal and coordinated functioning of each evolutionary level within the body—
evolutionary homeostasis. We can understand disease as a
breakdown in the functioning of one or more of these levels. Our
framework also gives us a new way to classify and discuss human
diseases.

This chapter will present an overview of human health from an
evolutionary perspective. It will deal with the human organism in
broad terms, and it starts far earlier than standard treatments of
human evolution. In fact, it starts at the beginning—the origin of
all life. Table 1 sets out 17 stages of human evolutionary health
that will be our guide for understanding human disease, pathology,
and medical problems. But before we start our evolutionary journey through the history of human health, we must be aware of the
agent of evolutionary fortune.

The theory of evolution by natural selection was first discovered by Charles Darwin and Alfred Russel Wallace, two 19th-
century English naturalists exposed at early ages by world travel to
the diversity of life around the globe. It is a no-nonsense theory
that explains so much, and so it is universally accepted by the
world's scientists. Darwin's 1859 book *The Origin of Species* is a
beautifully written, albeit somewhat lengthy, argument for evolution by natural selection. Evolutionary biologist Ernst Mayr has
recently succinctly outlined Darwin's argument into five basic facts
and three inferences.[1] From the first three facts (populations can
always increase more rapidly than their resources, populations tend
to stay the same size, and resources are always limited), Darwin
inferred that there will always be a struggle for existence among
individuals within populations (Inference Number One). From
Facts Three and Four (individuals are unique, and much of individual uniqueness is inherited), Darwin deduced (Inference Number Two) that in each generation there would be differential
survival and reproduction (the "survival of the fittest," to use Herbert Spencer's term). Here it is important to stress the reproduction part of the argument, because survival means nothing to

evolution unless the number of offspring is affected. Finally, evolution occurs when, generation after generation, differential reproduction leads to an eventual change in the population's inherited
characteristics (Inference Number Three). The characteristics may
be observable at the biochemical, genetic, physical, or behavioral
levels. With the discovery of the gene, which Darwin did not know
about, we now say that evolution occurs when gene frequencies in
a population change.

The Levels of Human Evolution

"Human evolution" is a term frequently used to mean just that little
bit of evolution from the last common ancestor of great apes, those
primates with whom we share some 98 percent of our genome, to
ourselves. But in this book we will take the long view. Human evolution entails all the steps in our lineage back to the primordial seas.
This scale of our purview is necessary because many aspects of our
biology, important to medicine, are much earlier adaptations than just
our evolutionary history since the ape-human split. Yet they have all
been incorporated into the functioning whole of a living human
being. Table 1 summarizes the 17 levels of human evolution used in
this book and serves as a framework for our further discussion.

Ground Zero—before Life Began

Earth coalesced some 5.2 billion years ago (5.2×10^9 years ago)
from swirling gases as the solar system formed around the Sun.
Earth, the third planet from the Sun, cooled down enough for
water (composed of hydrogen and oxygen) to form in a liquid state,
but it remained warm enough to prevent water from freezing.
Oceans formed in the depressions on Earth's crust. It was here, in
a "primordial soup," that the first stirrings of life began. Other elements necessary for life as we know it, such as carbon, nitrogen,
and many trace elements, were found in abundance on the early
Earth. To this day we require certain key elements for optimum
health, such as iron, manganese, copper, and cobalt, whose need

Table 1. Evolutionary Levels of **Human Structure and Function**

Level	Structural Organization	Function	Time (Years Ago)[1]	Embryonic Stage[2]	Homologues/Stage Relatives
0—Prebiotic	Elemental, molecular	Organic chemical reaction, chain elongation	$5.2–3.8 \times 10^9$	N.A.[3]	Oxygen, carbon, nitrogen, NH_3, H_2O, C_2HO_3, amino acids
1—Prokaryotes	Cell membrane, RNA, ATP, metabolic enzymes	Anaerobic metabolism, glycolysis, mitosis, actin contraction, cell membrane transport	$3.8–1.8 \times 10^9$	N.A. [4]	Archaeobacteria, Escherischia coli, Bacillus, cyanobacteria, spirochetes, Daptobacter
2—Unicellular eukaryotes	Nuclear membrane, DNA, cytochrome C, microtubules, mitochondria, lysosomes, G proteins	Aerobic metabolism, respiration, meiosis, DNA repair, sexual reproduction, nuclear membrane transport	$1.8–1.6 \times 10^9$	1	Amoebas, Paramecium, Euglenia

(Continued)

Table 1 (continued)

Level	Structural Organization	Function	Time (Years Ago)[1]	Embryonic Stage[2]	Homologues/ Stage Relatives
3—Morula	Aggregated totipotential cells, primitive hormones, extracellular matrix	Cell-to-cell interaction, induction	$1.6–1.5 \times 10^9$	2	Sponges
4—Blastocyst	Differentiated trophic and somatic cells, 2 germ layers	Cell specialization	$1.5–1.2 \times 10^9$	3–5	Choanoflagellates, fungi, plants
5—Animals	Muscle, nerve, and circulatory cells; phagocytes; blood; 2-chambered heart; homeotic genes; locomotor structures; mouth; cloaca; 3 germ layers	Copulation, active movement, natural immunity, inhibition of cell growth by compaction, gamete production, epithelial respiration, advanced hormone stimulation	$1.2–1.0 \times 10^9$	6–7 and gametogenesis	Worms, arthropods, mollusks, echinoderms

6—Chordates	Notochord, cartilage, somites and body segments, dorsal nerve cord, pharyngeal arches, tail, bilateral symmetry, endoskeleton	Gill respiration, sinusoidal muscle contraction for movement, neurotransmitter release; blood isotonic with seawater	1.0×10^9– 7.5×10^8	8–11	Sea squirt, lancelet (*Amphioxus*)
7A— Cartilaginous fish	Eye, liver, kidneys, suprarenal glands, inner ear, and limbs	Hearing, sense of balance, eggs laid in water, glucocorticoid hormones, immunoglobins (IgG)	7.5–4.5×10^8	12–14	Sharks, rays
7B—Bony fish	Sensory hair cells (cranial nerve 8), bony cranium and skeleton, teeth, swim bladder	Body support by fleshy fins, salt resorption by kidney, IgM, aldosterone	4.5–3.6×10^8	15	Coelacanth, zebra fish
8—Amphibians	Lung, limbs, NK cells, 3-chambered heart	Air breathing, cell-mediated immunity, "crawling"	3.6–3.0×10^8	16	Frog, salamander

(Continued)

Table 1 (*continued*)

Level	Structural Organization	Function	Time (Years Ago)[1]	Embryonic Stage[2]	Homologues/Stage Relatives
9—Reptiles	R-complex (brain), penis, vagina, gonads, advanced kidney, T and B lymphocytes	Broad cell-mediated immunity, water resorption by kidney, amniote egg, dry skin	$3.0–2.0 \times 10^8$	19–20	Lizard, snake, Komodo dragon
10—Mammals	Paleomammalian brain, 4-chambered heart, homeothermy, hair, lymph nodes, 7–8 Ig's, placenta, external ears, mandible, middle ear ossicles, differentiated teeth, breasts	Warm-bloodedness, very broad cell-mediated immune function, "creeping," nursing infants, reproduction in litters, insectivorous	2.0×10^8– 6.5×10^7	21–23 and fetal period	Monotremes—platypus, echidna; marsupials—opossums; placentals—tree shrews, rats, guinea pigs
11—Plesiadapiform primates	Neomammalian brain (simple), broad molar teeth	Arboreal, omnivorous, small litters	$6.5–5.6 \times 10^7$	Fetal period	Extinct, basal primates such as *Plesiadapis*

12—Prosimian primates	Orbital frontality, scent glands, nails on digits, hemochorial placenta, advanced ear structure	Stereoscopic and color vision, increased plants/fruits in diet, vertical clinging and leaping	$5.6–4.8 \times 10^7$	Fetal period	Tarsiers, lemurs, galagos, and lorises, as well as numerous extinct prosimians (*Notharctus* and *Smilodectes*)
13A—Anthropoids	Post-orbital bar in skull, deep mandibular body fused in midline	Decreased reliance on olfaction, L-gulonolactone oxidase deficiency	$4.8–2.3 \times 10^7$	Fetal period	New World monkeys, extinct late Eocene and Oligocene Old World anthropoids
13B—Old World anthropoids	2 premolars, marked sexual dimorphism (males larger), increased overall body size	Polygynous mating structure, increased internal competition for females, arboreal climbing, alcohol dehydrogenase	$3.7–2.3 \times 10^7$	Fetal period	Old World monkeys (macaques, baboons, langurs); extinct Oligocene anthropoids (*Aegyptopithecus*)

(Continued)

Table 1 (continued)

Level	Structural Organization	Function	Time (Years Ago)[1]	Embryonic Stage[2]	Homologues/ Stage Relatives
14—Hominoids	Enlarged brain, loss of tail, shoulder mobility	Arboreal hanging and brachiation, ability to use symbols, increased fat storage, loss of urate oxidase	2.3×10^7– 6.0×10^6	Fetal period	Lesser apes (gibbon and siamang), great apes (orangutan, chimpanzee, bonobo, and gorilla), extinct Miocene apes (*Proconsul*)
15—Hominids	Bipedalism, very enlarged brain, pelvic outlet same diameter as fetal head, spinal curves, molar teeth large compared to body size ("megamylic") and thick-enameled	Open and dry habitat, toolmaking and language ability, increased rate of brain glucose metabolism, dietary catholicism, manual dexterity	6.0×10^6– 5.0×10^5	Fetal period	Australopithecines, early *Homo* (*H. habilis* and *H. erectus*)
16—Humans	Neo-mammalian brain (complex), large body size, decreased molar size, barrel-shaped thorax	Omnivory and cooking, increased life span, advanced language and fully lateralized cerebral functions, elaborated liver P-450 detoxifying enzymes	2.5×10^6– 4.0×10^4	Fetal period	*Homo sapiens* and archaic relatives (*H. heidelbergensis* and Neandertals)

| 17—Human subgroups | Skin color differences, body proportion adaptations to climate, decreased size of dentition | Increased alcohol dehydrogenase activity, lactase, sickle cell trait, G6PD, occasional very high population densities, reliance on agriculture and restricted dietary range | 4.0×10^4– present | Fetal period | Human populations ("races")[5] |

[1] Ages follow Schopf, J.W. (ed.) 1983 Earth's Earliest Biosphere. Princeton Univ. Press, and Bengtson, S. (ed.) 1994 Early Life of Earth. New York: Columbia Univ. Press; Wang, D.Y.-C., S. Kumar, and S.B. Hedges 1999 Divergence time estimates for the early history of animal phyla and the origin of plants, animals, and fungi. Proc. Roy. Soc. London B 266:163-171; and Kumar, S., and S.B. Hedges 1998 A molecular timescale for vertebrate evolution. Nature 392:917-920; and Kay, R.F., C.F. Ross, and B.A. Williams 1997 Rethinking anthropoid origins. Science 275:797-804.

[2] Stages of embryonic development are sometimes referred to as "Carnegie stages" and follow O'Rahilly, R.O., and F. Müller 1996 Human Embryology and Teratology, 2nd ed. New York: Wiley-Liss.

[3] Stage 0 is the ground state of matter in the universe and thus is pre-existing to either organic life in general or our own individual life.

[4] Embryogenesis in eukaryotes does not recapitulate a prokaryote stage of cellular organization, although the stage of fertilization of the ovum by the sperm in which two pronuclei begin fusion and lack a single nuclear membrane may be homologous to a brief prokaryote-like phase of eukaryotic development. However, sex cells (eggs and sperms) are alive before conception and will stay alive after death–recombined in offspring–so they are, in a sense, "immortal" and part of our continuous connection to the rest of life on earth.

[5] Human populations are groups of *Homo sapiens* within which there is greater gene flow among individuals than there is with other groups. They are geographically delimited, and as such they can be termed biological "races", although this term has been widely misused. It is not synonymous with "ethnic group," does not imply any cultural, linguistic, religious, or political identity, is not accurately reflected by skin color, and populational differences do not imply superiority or inferiority. Population affinities of patients can, however, be important in susceptibility to disease and in effectiveness of specific medical therapies.

can only be explained by the still vaguely known chemical interactions of the nonliving molecules that ultimately gave rise to life.

We can look at this beginning stage of our evolution as the
inorganic chemistry of prelife, the period when the naked attributes of the molecules in the rocks and seas of the primordial Earth
were the prime actors on stage. How do we visualize the entities
that were ancestral to us at this time? Certainly, they were microscopic actors. Some theorists on the origin of life have called the
molecules "naked DNA," but they could equally well have been,
and probably were, a related molecule, RNA.[2] Today, RNA in our
bodies requires enzymes, specialized chemical catalysts in our cells
that speed up chemical reactions, in order to replicate itself. But on
the early Earth, it is likely that the pace of chemical change and
replication was much slower than it is today. In the early history of
life, RNA possessed enzymatic functions, which cause chemical
reactions to proceed more rapidly than normal. Natural selection
would have favored molecules of larger size because they could better resist the breaking up of chemical bonds by ultraviolet light or
mechanical current action. Thus they lasted longer and, self-
replicating, passed on their characteristics to a larger proportion of
succeeding molecules, including DNA.

Evolution of the First Cells

When naked DNA wrapped itself in a protective membrane, the
first cells, bacteria-like prokaryotes, were evolved. They developed
a process of organized cell division called "mitosis" that allowed a
cell to split into two, carrying a full complement of DNA into each
daughter cell. Each daughter cell was a clone—exactly identical to
its parent cell. They lived on primary elements, developing a
metabolism that required only sunlight, minerals, and amino acids.
The DNA message was translated into proteins in small units of
the cell called "ribosomes." Oxygen was poisonous to the early
prokaryotes. Advanced prokaryotes first evolved the ability to
break down simple sugars made by other prokaryotes and thus
brought in the innovation of glycolysis—still the biochemical basis
of our metabolic breakdown of food molecules. The citric acid
cycle, the central engine of the synthetic metabolism of aerobic

life, evolved to take in carbon dioxide to the cell and make bio-chemical precursors to all the body's amino acids, sugars, and lipids.[3] Some of the more advanced prokaryotes evolved whiplike waving cells on their cell walls to allow them to actively move through the water.

Some time in the murky depths of Archean time, stripped-down, parasitic organisms known as "viruses" evolved. Viruses have the ability to get through the prokaryote's cell membrane, insert themselves into the DNA, and take over the cell's repro-ductive machinery to make many more copies of themselves. This process kills the prokaryote, but there is also an unexpected bene-fit from an evolutionary perspective. Viruses move genetic material around, transferring genes from one cell that they have infected to another, thus creating genetic diversity—the raw material of nat-ural selection. Genetic experiments undertaken by viruses are an ancient heritage of our cells and probably have been important at many stages of our evolutionary history.[4]

The prokaryote stage of our evolution is Level 1 in our classifi-cation of human evolutionary levels—where life can be said to have begun—some 3.8 billion years ago based on combined pale-ontological and molecular studies (see Table 1). Today, when our dividing cells fail in their basic prokaryotic reproductive function and incorrectly parcel out their DNA to daughter cells, we have a mutation. Genetic mutations underlie or are associated with many birth defects (chapter 3) and cancers (chapter 5). And when our body ceases its basic prokaryotic functions of metabolism and cel-lular reproduction, we die (senescence and death are discussed in chapter 14).

The eukaryotes (Level 2) evolved a cell nucleus between 1.6 and 1.8 billion years ago, perhaps to more fully insulate their all-important DNA from the environment and to protect it from viral invasion. The eukaryote nucleus is much like a fortified castle, sur-rounded by a moat of cytoplasm, in turn protected by the outer wall of the cell membrane. A drawbridge—the "endoplasmic retic-ulum" (Latin for "that which retains within the plasma")—evolved to allow molecular foot traffic to cross the moat. The "rough" part of the endoplasmic reticulum (so named because this part of the membrane appears pebbly and irregular under the microscope) became the place where the protein-translating ribosomes nested in the eukaryote cell. A number of previously independent bacterial species evolved to live in the eukaryote moat—outside the nuclear castle walls but still protected by the outer perimeter of defenses. In return, they provided services to the cell. Oxygen-tolerant bacteria were incorporated into the cytoplasm as mitochondria—still today the organelles in which oxygen metabolism takes place in our cells. Other oxygen-tolerant bacteria were incorporated into the cytoplasm as "lysosomes." These organelles stored and released caustic nitrite bleach, wiping out invaders breeching the cell's outer perimeter. Another kind of prokaryote, capable of movement, was incorporated within the cell to move things around inside the cell, as well as to move the cell itself by waving on the outside of the cell. These prokaryotes were the "microtubules."[5]

Among the most important jobs of the microtubules was to pull long DNA segments called "chromosomes" apart in the new eukaryote method of reproduction—sex. Microtubules attach to one of each of a pair of chromosomes and pull them to opposite sides of the cell in preparation for cell division. This process, meiosis, reduces the amount of DNA in a daughter cell to one half, effecting a 50–50 split of a cell's genes, and allows eukaryotes to produce sex cells for later recombination into a new individual with a unique genetic makeup. Mistakes in meiosis can have a profound effect on our development. For example, if our chromosome 21 does not properly separate from its partner, the resulting sex cell (a sperm or an egg with an extra chromosome 21) can recombine during sexual reproduction to form a Down's syndrome child.

Around 1.5 billion years ago, eukaryote cells discovered that there was safety in numbers. Molecular studies indicate that this is the date of the evolutionary divergence of the plants, animals, and fungi.[6] Fossil aggregates of cells found in Australia, South Africa, and Canada show that by at least 850 million years ago the eukaryote cells had bonded together—circling the wagons for protection and defense. Cells adapted to interact with one another, producing proteins whose functions were to signal from one cell to another—the first hormones. Among the signals that one cell sent to another were the commands to start or stop duplication. Cell-to-cell interactions are involved in many disease processes that we will discuss because cells had to overcome their defensive adaptations in order to live together in a colony of cells that we call an "organism." The morula, the mulberry-shaped ball of embryonic cells that develops shortly after conception, is homologous to this evolutionary stage, called here Level 3. There are no known living examples of Level 3 organisms on Earth today, having presumably been outcompeted long ago by more advanced multicellular organisms.

Level 4 occurs when the ball of cells organizes into two populations of cells—one destined to become a body and one destined to become the feeding mechanism. There is no clear fossil evidence for this stage of evolutionary development, the "blastocyst," but it is fundamental to the development of all multicellular organisms alive today. It occurs when a space opens up in the cells of the morula that will eventually become the lumen of our gastrointestinal tract. Level 4 is a focus of intense research in developmental biology and genetics because here genetic modifiers evolved that allow genes to cooperate in forming multicellular organisms.[7] It is at Level 4 that our ancestry diverges from that of plants, explaining (because of our shared ancestry) why plant poisons may also harm us. Our last common ancestor with fungi also dates from this time, a fact that explains why an antibacterial substance discovered by Alexander Fleming in 1928 and named by him "penicillin" kills bacteria and not us. Marine organisms called "choanoflagellates," only now becoming known, are living relatives of this ancient ancestor.[8]

The First Animals

The two-layered structure of a blastocyst in Level 4 gives rise to a three-layered sandwich of cells characteristic of the first truly active organisms—animals. The transformation from microscopic, three-layered[9] embryonic disk to a body form observable to the naked eye recapitulates an ancient evolutionary progression every generation. It is no less miraculous for its repetitiousness. A complex pattern of folding along both the long axis and the sides of the embryo occurs to form a body wall that encloses the internal organs. The human embryo folds toward its center like a swimming jellyfish, converging onto its future navel.

As the embryo folds, a series of transverse strips of tissue known as "somites" forms along its length from front to back. They account for such serially homologous structures as insect segments, fish gills, and human ribs and are under the control of homeotic genes. These genes were formed by genetic mutation, having been duplicated from a previous segment of DNA. Edward Lewis discovered homeotic genes in the fruit fly, and won the Nobel Prize for this discovery in 1995. We share this pattern of homeotic development with such animals as fruit flies, zebra fish, and mice—all objects of very active current research in developmental biology. Problems with homeotic genes or the playing out of their developmental messages are at the base of a number of birth defects and disruptive effects of chemical toxins during development.

With the evolution of body size visible to the naked eye, animals develop from a large colony into an empire of cells. Cells in animals become specialized and organize into aggregates of similar cells called "organs." Cells need to communicate with other cells in the same organ, as well as with cells in distant parts of the empire. Two basic adaptations appear in animals to accomplish these tasks—hormones and nerves.

Cells become adapted to producing and releasing complexly folded biochemicals specific to an internal environment within the cell that is distributed to other cells by the courier system of the body, the circulation. Certain cells have specially adapted "catchers" for these hormones called "receptors." The receptors bind to the hormones at the cell surface and then send "second messenger" molecules inside to cause predetermined reactions within the cell. All endocrine diseases of modern humanity are basically Level 5 problems—either an inability of the originating organ to throw the correct hormonal pass or of the target organ to catch it.

Nerves are more advanced methods of hard-wiring the body for action. Nerve cells evolved in the first animals in order to conduct information directly from one site to another. Nerves thus do not broadcast their messages to all cells in the body. They have a discrete origin and end point, and they must have a point of connection—a synapse—with another cell in order to deliver their message. The fossil evidence for this stage of our evolution is a blank, and we deduce much of the history of adaptations from comparisons with modern invertebrates with which we share our Level 5 ancestors. Primitive sight and smell first evolved during this time.

The first fossil evidence for the next stage of our animal evolution (Level 6) comes from the Burgess Shale of British Columbia, Canada, dating to between 530 and 550 million years ago and discovered by Charles Doolittle Walcott in 1909.[10] A single, mushy-bodied, elongate, and bilaterally symmetrical species named *Pikaia* lived among the many primitive invertebrate species that abounded in these ancient seas. It was the first chordate—an animal with a rod of cartilage, the notochord, along its back to help it flex from side to side in swimming along the seafloor. The notochord came to form parts of our spinal column. Among the medically relevant aspects of Level 6 is a remnant of the notochord, the so-called nucleus pulposus, forming the central part of our intervertebral disks. This is the part that "slips" in a slipped disk, pressing on a spinal nerve and causing excruciating back pain.

During this time, the olfactory nerve (our first cranial nerve), with which we still smell, evolved to connect specialized aroma-sensing cells in the nose region to other nerves in the primitive brain that control the muscles of the body. When our Level 6 ancestor smelled something good to eat, it moved in that direction. Other senses that became more advanced in function during this time were sight, mediated by the optic nerve (cranial nerve two) to the retina and the oculomotor nerve (cranial nerve three), which moved the eye around; taste, sensations from the mouth region sent to the brain by cranial nerves seven, eight, and nine; balance, information about the position of the body in relation to gravity made necessary because the animal could now actively move; and vibratory sense, used by the animal to detect the rapid movement or rush of water made by a predator about to eat it. Body balance and vibratory sense, a primitive sense of hearing, are both functions of cranial nerve eight. These adaptations are 750 million to a billion years old. Blindness, hearing loss, and vertigo are perturbations of Level 6 adaptations.

Origins of the Vertebrates

Our first vertebrate ancestors were fish (Level 7). We spent an astounding 390 million years of our evolution as fish—first as primitive, jawless, cartilaginous, sharklike forms, and then later as bony fish with true jaws and skeletons. We left the fish stage some 360 million years ago, but it is sobering to contemplate that we have spent more of our evolution as fish than as land-living tetrapods. Much of our basic anatomy and physiology remains fishy—our eyes, liver, kidneys, suprarenal (adrenal) glands, cranium, ears, and limbs all evolved first in our fish ancestors. We still hear through an ancient gill slit, and we still use many of the same hormones, such as aldosterone (produced by our kidneys) and cortisol (produced by the suprarenal glands). Immunoglobulin G, the mainstay of our immune system, first evolved in fish and still protects us today. When our limbs fail to develop the individual elements and digits of fingers and toes, and a child is born with paddle-shaped appendages, it is a Level 7 phenomenon.

Lobe-finned fish like the living-fossil crossopterygian fish, the coelacanth, native to the deep sea around Madagascar and Indonesia, are similar to our ancestors who crawled up out of the water onto land. Lobe-fins were ancestral to the first amphibians (Level 8), animals known as labyrinthodonts that flourished 325 million years ago and which could live in both water and air. These early amphibians are familiar as the "legged fish" anticreationist logos seen on American car bumpers. They represent our common ancestry with the salamanders, the toads, and the frogs.

The swim bladder, first used by fish to equilibrate themselves in water, evolved in the amphibians to become a site of oxygen exchange in the body—our future lungs. When emphysema renders our lungs capable of only partial oxygen exchange, we have essentially reverted to an amphibian level of functioning. The fleshy fins became sturdier and longer, but they still splayed out widely when the amphibians wriggled across dry land. Our five-fingered hand (much more primitive than our foot structure) is inherited from our amphibian forebears.

Reptiles (Level 9) evolved from the amphibians and became much more fully adapted to life on land. Our ancestors were the early and primitive mammal-like reptiles. The paleontologist

Alfred Romer once described these creatures as an odd mix between a lizard and a dog. Their primary reproductive adaptation was the leathery amniote egg (the amnion is a layer inside the egg that stores wastes and allows the egg to "breathe" through its shell). But not only was the amniote egg, unlike amphibian eggs, laid on land, it was also already fertilized. Reptiles evolved copulation and the anatomy that goes along with it. Male reptiles have an intromissive organ, a penis, that introduces sperm into the female's vagina for internal fertilization. No longer could aquatic predators dine on the caviar of our ancestors. The brain evolved along with the more intricate behavior patterns associated with mating, territorial defense, and maintaining social hierarchies. The teeth of the mammal-like reptiles differentiated into front-biting and puncturing teeth, while the back teeth adopted more slicing and grinding functions. Their skin grew thicker and impervious to drying out, unlike amphibians. And their limbs evolved to be longer and stronger and able to carry them along without dragging their belly on the ground. Kidneys evolved long tubules to reabsorb water from urine and thus prevent dehydration on land.

Our mammal-like reptile ancestors were successful for 100 million years. They gave rise not only to the early mammals, our ancestors, but to two groups of descendants originally much more successful than ourselves—the dinosaurs and the birds. Fred Flintstone notwithstanding, we were small and insignificant creatures when our giant reptile cousins held sway over Earth.

Mammal and Primate Levels of Our Evolution

The first mammals (Level 10) were small, active, and unobtrusive animals that scurried around on the forest floor. They may have been similar to an opossum. They had a relatively larger brain than their reptile ancestors, developing those brain centers especially important in emotions known as the limbic system, but they still relied heavily on their sense of smell. Mammals have fully differentiated teeth—incisors, canines, premolars, and molars—an adaptation that allows more efficient obtaining and processing of food. Early mammals may have been nocturnal, and evolved a high metabolism—warm-bloodedness—possibly to offset the low night-time temperatures. It may have been this adaptation that allowed them to survive the climatic deterioration that did in the dinosaurs.

Mammals took protection of offspring to extremes. Not only did they keep the innovation of reptilian copulation, ensuring that parental sex cells came directly into contact, but the more advanced mammals, the pouched marsupials and the placental mammals, did away with egg laying altogether. The fertilized egg develops inside the mother, safely nurtured within a specialized organ called the "uterus." When an offspring is finally born, it is ready to run about on its own. There is no period of unhatched helplessness during which ovivorous predators could eat an entire clutch of offspring. After birth, mammalian mothers nurse their offspring from specialized sweat glands that secrete a nutritious and infection-fighting fluid called "milk."

Female mammals have breasts for nursing, and a sophisticated reproductive anatomical adaptation that males never have—the placenta. The placenta grows partly from the embryo and partly from the mother. It serves as a lifeline attaching the developing embryo to the wall of the mother's uterus. A four-chambered heart in mammals efficiently separates oxygenated blood returning via the pulmonary veins from the lungs and deoxygenated blood returning from the body via the venae cavae. This is the adaptation that not only allows a higher metabolic turnover of oxygen and mammalian homeothermy (warm-bloodedness), but also gives a mammalian mother the excess oxygenation potential to "breathe" for her developing fetus. New hormonal adaptations evolved to monitor a more finely tuned reproductive and metabolic physiology. Breast cancer, many heart defects, and an overactive thyroid gland are problems with our mammalian level of organization.

The transition from generalized mammal to primitive primate (Level 11) is mostly one of degree rather than qualitative change. The first primates were small plesiadapiforms,[11] and they appear in the fossil record soon after the demise of the dinosaurs. The primates became adapted to living in trees, perhaps to avoid most ground-living predators. Their limbs were adapted to grasping, still a basic human trait, at least as regards our hands.

Early primates would have resembled an intelligent squirrel or a tree shrew (a small insectivore that still lives in the forests of southeastern Asia). Their brain, however, was relatively larger and more advanced, with greater development of cerebral areas, particularly the part concerned with vision. Primates were becoming visual animals. Our plesiadapiform ancestors were likely active in the daytime, trading the ancient security of blanketing darkness for a vantage point of inaccessibility in the trees. It is likely that our primordial fears of heights, the dark, and snakes trace back to our early primate adaptations to life in the trees. Another little reminder of our plesiadapiform ancestry is the presence of little "mittens" of enamel along the biting edge of children's recently erupted upper central incisor teeth, recalling the fusion of primitive front teeth cones into wide, nipping incisors.

Prosimian primates (Level 12) were still small creatures, still living in trees, but they represent a major advance over the preceding basal primates. Claws evolved into flat nails to support fleshy finger- and toetips that were well adapted to grabbing onto branches and climbing. Fingerprint patterns and sweaty palms— adaptations to increase security of grip—trace to this level of our evolution. When your hands start to sweat before you go onstage, you are really reliving the preparatory stage of a prosimian leap of faith.

Our eyes at the prosimian stage of evolution moved forward on the skull to focus overlapping images on our retinas, giving us stereoscopic vision, better depth perception, more accurate jumping in the trees, and better prey-catching ability.[12] Color vision also evolved during this time, imparting the ability to tell ripe plant foods from unripe, even at a distance. As our prosimian ancestors gained visual acuity and depth perception, they lost the range of peripheral vision so important to most other mammals in alerting them to predator attacks. Comparative primate behavior and functional anatomy both indicate that prosimians evolved an increasingly complex social organization at this time to ensure that trusted relatives and group members were watching their backs. Advanced prosimians (sometimes termed "haplorhines," a group including tarsiers and higher primates), perhaps because they ate so much fruit, lost the ability to synthesize vitamin C, regaining some metabolic

energy as they did so.[13] Scurvy, a deficiency disease of vitamin C, is
thus a Level 12 malady. Prosimians still retained use of the sense of
smell in their social interactions—marking territory with scent
glands located on the forearms and near the anus, as well as by uri-
nating. Our use of perfumes, colognes, aftershave, and scented
shampoos represents an ancient prosimian legacy; our use of toilets
and deodorants, our fight against it. Sebaceous cysts on the front
parts of our forearms and near our anus are remnants of ancient
prosimian scent glands that can become inflamed and painful,
requiring surgical removal.

In common parlance, the terms "monkey" and "ape" are frequently used interchangeably. In primate taxonomy, however,
these two terms are quite specific. Monkeys are generally smaller,
have a slightly smaller relative brain size, have a tail, and run on all
fours, either along the ground or along branches of trees (with
their hands palm downward). Barbary "apes" (actually macaques),
baboons (even though they lack a tail), and spider monkeys
(although they can swing through trees) are all monkeys. Apes are
generally bigger, smarter, tailless, able to hang under a tree limb
(an ability termed "brachiation"), and, when quadrupedal, support
their weight on the fingers of an incurved hand (in knuckle-
walking or fist-walking). The great apes are the African gorilla and
chimpanzee (including the pygmy chimp, or bonobo) and the
Asian orangutan. The lesser apes are the Asian gibbon and sia-
mang.

Although it is technically true that we "did not evolve from a
monkey," we do share an anthropoid ancestry with the monkeys
(Level 13). At a site in northern Egypt called the Fayum, fossils preserve monkeylike tailed primates close to our ancestry. These include
such species as Catopithecus and Aegyptopithecus, discovered by Elwyn
Simons.[14] Darwin was fascinated with human children born with
tails, an "atavism" which he hypothesized recalled an earlier stage of
evolution.[15] We can now say that such children have an evolutionary Level 13 retention, one that is easily corrected by surgery.

Our hominoid ancestors are known from early Miocene sites in
equatorial Africa dating to 23 to 18 million years ago. These were
the proconsulids—tailless climbing apes with feet that could grasp
onto branches as well as their hands could. When modern humans'
feet collapse inward with a hypermobile big toe, a condition that

we call "flatfeet," it is a reversion to the ancestral hominoid condition of Level 14. In the middle Miocene, the hominoids underwent several genetic mutations that allowed them to conserve
water in a desiccating landscape by excreting uric acid (see chapter 10). In the process, however, they predisposed themselves to a
painful buildup of uric acid crystals in their joints called "gout," a
Level 14 disease.

Hominid Evolution

Sometime about 5 to 7 million years ago, human ancestors came
down from the trees, probably because the trees were thinning out
as climates became drier.[16] The defining characteristic of these
African terrestrial hominoids, known as "hominids," was walking
around on two legs. Bipedalism at first appears to be a very unusual
adaptation for getting around. But gibbons, our lesser-ape, tree-
swinging cousins, are also bipedal when they come to the ground
(which is rarely), and an entire order of vertebrates, the birds, are
primarily bipedal when they are not flying. But hominids are one
of the only animals to adopt bipedalism as their primary mode of
progression. As hominids evolved larger body size through time,
they also were beset by a number of structural problems unique to
a bipedal animal—slipped vertebral disks, hernias, and back
pain—which are discussed in chapter 11.

The primary adaptation of hominids is the enlarged brain,
which became expanded over that of apes among the australopithecines, a group of African hominids dating back to about 4
million years ago. The australopithecines could make and use
simple bone and wood tools, as new research has shown, but they
almost certainly could not speak as we do. An example of a
hominid Level 15 disorder is Broca's aphasia, an inability to form
words.

Early species of the genus *Homo* appear about 2.5 million years
ago, bringing with them the first stone tools, bigger body size, and
an even larger brain. The brain becomes so large in fact that fitting
a fetus's head through the mother's pelvis at birth is difficult. Many
of the obstetric problems and fetal distress that may accompany
human birth are Level 16 issues.[17]

Human diet completed most of its long evolution during Level
15. Archaeological remains show that early humans ate meat—
both scavenged and occasionally hunted. Plant foods, however,
remained important parts of the diet. Fire was an innovation that
came along some 1.6 million years ago, and allowed our ancestors to
cook, soften up, and detoxify many previously inedible plant foods.
Our teeth, from the times of *Homo habilis* to *Homo erectus* and
finally to *Homo sapiens*, have consistently decreased in size as we
have coevolved with stone tools and fire. The degradation of our
diet, and the many diseases of modern civilization that are associated with it, are primarily dysfunctions of our Level 16 adaptations.

Modern human evolution—the biological changes that have
occurred within the past 40,000 years—constitutes the most recent
level in our evolutionary framework, Level 17. All human populations in the world today, sometimes termed "races," are members of
the same species, *Homo sapiens*. They may differ in body proportions, skin color, hair form, skull features, gene percentages, and
minor biochemical traits. These differences, however, may be
important to aspects of peoples' health, and thus are of interest to
us here. For example, sickle-cell genes (causing sickle-cell anemia
when inherited from both parents) evolved in African populations
as a defense against malarial disease, and cystic fibrosis genes (causing cystic fibrosis when inherited from both parents) evolved in
European populations as a defense against cholera.

Ten thousand years ago, or much later in many parts of the
world, modern humans learned to bring previously wild plants and
animal species under domestication. The so-called Agricultural
Revolution provided a more predictable source of food, allowed
village life, and created population centers where art and learning
could flourish. But there was also a precipitous drop in the variety
of plant and animal foods eaten, with an associated increase in
nutritional diseases, documented by a drop in peoples' mean
stature.[18] High population densities facilitated the more rapid
spread of infectious diseases.[19] In a real sense, almost all of the preventable diseases and illnesses associated with modern civilization
discussed in this book are by-products of Level 17 adaptations.

Level 17 is by far the shortest, temporally speaking, and the
only level less than a million years in length. It has also seen some
of the greatest change—the development of public health, sterile

medical procedures, antibiotics, anesthetics, and preventive medicine. Human beings now have the longest life expectancy of any time in our evolutionary history because ancient causes of death and morbidity—trauma, parasites, and infectious diseases—have been drastically reduced. Unlike the preceding evolutionary levels, Level 17 is also open-ended, subject to continuing evolution and change. We know that the diseases of civilization that now afflict us are not inevitable, because our ancestors and so many of our fellow modern *Homo sapiens* with technologically primitive lifestyles have avoided them. The optimistic message of evolutionary medicine is that our future health can be enhanced by applying these lessons learned from past human evolution. If we defeat the diseases of civilization, how much longer could we live? If we could live an extra 20 or 30 years, would we want to? Balancing the promise of longevity with the realities of senescence will be a topic to which we return in the final chapter.

3

An Evolutionary Child's Birthright: Perinatal and Pediatric Diseases

Childhood was the most dangerous time of life for most early hominids. Mortality was high, not only from predators, which prefer the weak, the young, and the inexperienced, but also from parasites and infectious diseases, which can overtake an immature immune system. Predation is no longer a worry for most of us, and modern antibiotics, public health measures, and Western medical practices have now drastically reduced the mortal effects of childhood diseases. This change in our demography—reduction of major childhood mortality—largely accounts for our increased life expectancy over our ancestors.

Modern childhood is, however, not a bed of roses for many. Mortality may be reduced, but morbidity—living with a reduced quality of life—is a significant factor for many millions of the world's children. This chapter is about preventing and reducing childhood morbidity by referring to evolutionary principles. Our story, naturally, begins at conception.

Ontogeny and Phylogeny—Haeckel's Insight

Our individual life begins, like all life has evolved, with a single cell (Level 1). Using a linear genetic code inherited from ancestors, a single cell develops according to a grand sequential plan. There are basic similarities between the evolution of life and the development (ontogeny) of an individual. With what we now know of genetics and evolution, this makes sense. Evolution builds on what came before—the genetic message that it is given by reproduction to work with. Code can be added or deleted from the genetic message as natural selection acts as editor each generation, but the basic plan stays the same. We, tomato plants, fruit flies, and kangaroos all develop into a ball of cells called a morula, which then differentiates into a three-layered disk, which then twists, turns, and curls in various ways to form a body. The closer the genetic relationship between two species, the more similar the details of the twisting and turning, as well as the final forms of the bodies. This is why studying comparative anatomy has provided us so much insight into the evolutionary relationships among organisms.

Ernst Haeckel, the great 19th-century Darwinian naturalist who developed the concepts of "ecology" and "phylogeny," coined the inimitable phrase "ontogeny recapitulates phylogeny"—in other words, the development of an individual restates its species' evolutionary history. This insight refers to the mind-bending concept that the development of each one of us from the single-celled zygote formed by the fusion of egg and sperm goes through largely the same organic transformations that whole species evolved through during the past billion and a half years. Some academic naysayers focusing on what was edited out, that is, the differences between evolutionary history and individual development, have missed the idea, but its basic validity has withstood synthesis with modern genetics and developmental biology. Although organisms actually recapitulate their ancestors' developmental stages (and not their adult anatomy), and the stages may be subject to alteration by later natural selection, Haeckel's evolutionary hypothesis remains one of the basic theoretical foundations of comparative anatomy and evolutionary biology.[1]

Haeckel's thesis is important to evolutionary medicine because it helps us to understand when, how, and why birth defects occur. Recalling the 17 adaptive levels from chapter 2, we can classify birth defects as failures to achieve the structural integrity of any one of those levels. In the birth defect in which a child is born with eyes on the sides, rather the front, of his or her face, a condition termed "ocular hypertelorism," there has been a failure to progress from Level 11 to Level 12, the prosimian to the anthropoid. In human evolution, this change happened some 45 million years ago. In human development, it happens between the fifth and eighth weeks after conception. In this particular trait, the child becomes stuck at the prosimian grade of organization. The skull of a child with ocular hypertelorism looks remarkably like that of an overgrown galago. Surgery can correct the wayward eye sockets and allow the child to develop normal eye function.

In whatever manner birth defects are caused—by either harmful substances crossing the placenta or by spontaneous genetic mutations—they often harken back to an earlier stage of our evolution. For example, when a baby is born with extra fingers, and there are more than one, there are frequently three. The discovery of an eight-toed fossil amphibian in Greenland a few years ago, one close to our ancestry, helps to explain that this malformation is a reversion to an earlier state still encoded in our genes. The more recently evolved genetic code that edited out those extra three fingers somehow was lost or not expressed in the malformed baby. In the scheme of evolutionary stages used in this book, this malformation is at Level 8. Table 2 lists the most common birth defects and places them in the scheme of evolutionary stages used in this book.

Classifying birth defects in this manner is new. The usefulness of such a scheme for directing future research has yet to be shown, but it is instructive to us in demonstrating that teratogens and mutagens do not act randomly. Rather, the monkey wrenches that the environment may throw into our genetic machinery disrupt development at particular and predictable places along our ontogenetic-phylogenetic continuum. When we have a more complete knowledge of the genetics of the birth defects, now a promising possibility with the sequencing of the human genome, a fuller and more specific picture of the evolutionary adaptations that we have will emerge. Preventing and treating birth defects will be an

Table 2. Common Human Birth Defects and the
Evolutionary Developmental Stages Affected

A normal human baby is a culmination of a sequence of developmental stages mirroring, in large part, evolutionary stages. The following illustrative birth defects are truncations of normal development at any one of the stages.

Birth Defect	Stage of Evolution	Explanation
Flipper limbs (syndactyly/meromelia)	7	Undifferentiated fingers and toes recall Silurian fish ancestors
Incomplete or absent septa between atria and ventricle	7	Reestablishment, to varying degrees, of a two-chambered heart characteristic of fish
Cleft palate	8	A deficiency, to varying degrees, of the hard palate first evolved in reptiles
Extra fingers (polydactyly)	8	Eight fingers and seven toes are characteristic of the Devonian labyrinthodont amphibians *Acanthostega* and *Ichthyostega*
Open spinal canal (spina bifida)	8	Lack of a complete dorsal arch of the vertebrae is a characteristic of the normal early amphibian skeleton
Incomplete or absent septum between the ventricles	8	A three-chambered heart similar to that of a frog; oxygenated blood from the lungs is mixed with deoxygenated blood and pumped to the body
Constriction (coarctation) of the aorta	9	Narrowing of the aorta on the left side, in addition to the right aorta (which disappears in mammals)
Extra breasts (polymastia)/ extra nipples (polythelia)	10	Multiple nipples and breasts are characteristic of nonprimate mammals
Smooth-fissured brain (lissencephaly)	10	Relatively unfissured cerebrum is early mammalian in form
Widely spaced eyes (ocular hypertelorism)	11	Widely separated eyes similar to Paleocene plesiadapid primates
"Waiter's tip hand" (Erb-Duchenne palsy)	15	Damage to the upper part of the brachial nerve plexus caused by its damage, made susceptible by the apelike lateral extension of the shoulder
Congenital wryneck (torticollis)	16	Condition brought about by birth trauma and affecting the unique human adaptation of keeping the head erect in bipedal posture

important part of the nascent field of molecular medicine, and human evolution will be at its center.

Birth Defects as Broken Links in the Chain of Being

Birth defects are horrific, inflicting gross anatomical deformations for life upon a newborn child. Until recently, embryologists referred to children with major birth defects as "monsters," and, indeed, the name of the field for the study of birth defects, "teratology," means just this. The terrible emotional effect of birth defects can first be seen in the transition of parents' emotions from eager anticipation prior to birth to shocked disbelief after the birth of a deformed baby. The guilt that many parents feel may be overwhelming, prompting them to consider what they could have done to prevent having a baby with a birth defect. Understanding the defect can be an important part in helping families cope with and emotionally come to terms with birth defects.

Disruptions in anatomical structure or physiological function occur when conditions fall outside the range of normality—the range of environments and activities that evolution has adapted our bodies to expect. Most common birth defects can be traced to exceeding normal conditions for prenatal development. Some of the defects are caused by exceeding the immediate range of needs of the developing embryo and fetus—effects that are termed "teratogenic"—and others are caused by genetic mistakes—effects that we can term "mutagenic."

The most well-known teratogen, a substance that causes birth defects, is thalidomide. This sedative and antinausea drug was introduced in Europe in the late 1950s after extensive tests on laboratory animals, in which it was found to be safe. But by the early 1960s German researchers realized that a spate of babies born with flipperlike arms and legs could be traced to their mothers' use of thalidomide during bouts of morning sickness when they had been pregnant. Thalidomide was found to derail development of the limb buds, a Level 7 to 8 adaptation in our classification, trapping a fetus in the fish stage of development. The limb buds develop from the body wall of the embryo during the third through the fifth weeks of development, and if the mother took thalidomide during this time, her baby had the defect, termed "phocomelia" ("seal limbs").[2] Unfortunately, very little can be done to correct the defect surgically because most of the limb structures simply did not develop.

The most common birth defect caused by a genetic mutation is Down's syndrome.[3] In this condition, a pair of number 21 chromosomes (the smallest), fails to migrate correctly to one of the parents' sex cells. When that double-21 sex cell merges with the other parent's normal sex cell, with one number 21 chromosome, the condition of trisomy 21 (Down's syndrome) results. A Down's syndrome child has the slanted eyes, mental retardation, and short stature that gave the condition the infelicitous name of Mongolian idiocy, now no longer used. Maternal age of greater than 40 years increases the chances of having a Down's syndrome child. Damage to the mother's sex cells from mutagens, the substances that cause genetic mutations, is thought to be the main cause. No similar condition is known in nonhuman primates or other animals.

It is significant that thalidomide does not cause defects in lab animals and yet is so devastating to developing human beings, and that Down's syndrome is a uniquely human defect. Human development apparently presents some significant differences from other animals. Evolutionary medicine helps to explain why the defects happen.

The Human Placenta and an Open Gate to Teratogens

The broad story of human evolution is really one of K-selection— the type of natural selection in which parents invest much effort in relatively fewer offspring. K-selected offspring are pampered, protected from predation and other environmental insults, while r-selected species' offspring have to sink or swim early on. Primates do not have litters of offspring like most other mammals. We humans, like the rest of the primates, have one or two babies at a time, and females have only two nipples for nursing. More than two young offspring just cannot be fed by primates in the natural state. After birth, primate parents within a social group expend tremendous energy protecting and feeding their young.

Humans and the anthropoid primates have extended the infant care theme into the womb. The nutrition that a human fetus receives via its mother's circulation is much richer than that of other mammals. The energy-rich sugar glucose is the primary food molecule, but many other substances of nutritive, immunological, and hormonal importance in the mother's body cross over to the fetus as well. A unique organ, the placenta, evolved in the mammals (Level 10) to move maternal nutrients to the fetus and to remove fetal metabolic wastes to the mother's bloodstream for elimination from her body.[4] The placenta also becomes an important endocrine organ, producing a number of essential hormones for both mother and fetus.

Physicians used to think of the placenta as a barrier, protecting the fetus from most if not all harmful substances in the mother's body. Thalidomide and subsequent research have changed all that. The human placenta is now recognized as a very efficient mechanism of cotransferring maternal and fetal substances. It is in large part so efficient in humans because it has become very thin. When a fertilized egg implants in the wall of the uterus, it begins to grow into the organ's muscular wall and becomes surrounded by growing uterine arteries. In humans and the higher primates, the end walls of the mother's arteries open up, pumping the mother's blood out of her body and into the placenta, delivering oxygen and nutrients and absorbing carbon dioxide and other wastes. But the blood entering the placenta does not cross the cellular wall of the embryo and, normally, there is never an actual mixing of maternal and fetal blood. Large-scale mixing of maternal blood with fetal blood is fatal to the fetus if it occurs. The single-celled wall of the fetal circulatory system acts as a membrane permitting osmosis between maternal blood and fetal blood. Only anthropoid primates have this very efficient, but potentially dangerous, "hemochorial" placenta.

No one knows exactly why rat babies do not develop meromelia when their mothers are administered thalidomide.[5] Rats, like most other mammals, have several tissue levels between maternal and fetal circulatory systems, and it stands to reason that the lower sensitivity to teratogens seen in nonprimate lab animals is largely due to this anatomical difference. What has evolved in humans as an extremely efficient mechanism for transferring nutrients can also deliver harmful substances from mother to fetus. The human placenta is an open gate to teratogens, making our world of synthetic chemicals, pharmaceuticals, and environmental toxins a dangerous place for the developing embryo. A number of known substances cause human birth defects, listed in Table 3. Some of the most common are caused by a mother's substance abuse—drinking, cocaine use, and smoking—and by disease transmitted from mother to fetus. Less clearly causative, but certainly contributory to birth defects, is poor maternal diet. Because of the heightened efficiency of our evolved reproductive biology, what happens to the mother happens, sometimes in magnified terms, to her unborn offspring.

Table 3. A Short List of Known Human Teratogenic Agents and the Birth Defects They Cause

Human Teratogen	Birth Defect(s)	Description of Effect
Thalidomide (anti-morning-sickness drug)	Meromelia	Limb buds poorly formed or lacking
Mercury	Minamata disease	Nervous system and musculoskeletal malformations
Ethyl alcohol	Fetal alcohol syndrome	Impairment of brain and nervous system/mental retardation; characteristic facial features
Hydantoin (antiepilepsy drug)	Fetal hydantoin syndrome	Impairment of brain and nervous system/mental retardation; characteristic facial features
Cocaine	"Crack baby" syndrome	Diffuse impairment of nervous system
Diethylstilbestrol (synthetic estrogen)	Clear cell carcinoma in female offspring	Cell proliferation in uterus or vagina
Erytretinoin (retinoic acid antiacne medication)	Vitamin A hyperosis	Malformations of nervous system, such as neural tube defect

Prevention of birth defects entails a mother avoiding the known teratogens and other potentially harmful substances, because her placenta will spoon-feed it all to her baby. Evolution has aided in the detection of teratogens. "Morning sickness" during the early stages of pregnancy is likely an evolved aversion to foods containing alkaloids that are potentially injurious to a developing embryo.[6] Animal tissues that could harbor parasites and other pathogens should also be avoided.[7] This was exactly the reaction that thalidomide was developed to overcome. But there are many, many other substances that cause birth defects and that are not deterred by the early warning system of morning sickness.

The Cumulative Effect of Mutagens

Mutations have been of interest to evolutionary scientists for many years because genetic innovations are the raw material of evolution. Without mutations there would be no source of new evolutionary adaptations. Unfortunately, most mutations are harmful. They occur at low but constant rates in any biological population. In the laboratory, many substances can cause mutations. In fact, almost any chemical or biologically active stimulus, if excessively concentrated, can cause them. Ammonia, mustard gas, X rays, ultraviolet light, and even oxygen can cause genetic changes. Cumulative effects of mutagens account for the mutation that causes Down's syndrome.

When mammals started to internalize their reproduction and retain their eggs within their bodies, a number of changes took place. External shells, to prevent water loss, were no longer needed. And eggs were produced and kept inside the body. In long-lived human beings, the eggs that are produced in the ovaries are formed before the birth of the woman who will release them one at a time at ovulation when she is an adult. Eggs ovulated after many years of sitting in the ovaries have been subjected to years of circulating mutagenic effects. Damage to the DNA of an egg of older mothers is thought to be the basic reason behind Down's syndrome and similar genetic defects. Down's syndrome is the most common because it affects the smallest chromosome, with the least amount of duplicated genetic information. Additions or deletions of larger chromosomes are usually fatal.

Genetic abnormalities and associated birth defects, such as Down's syndrome, are effects of the long human life span. People have a maximum life span of over 100 years, well above average for a mammal of our body size. As part of our increased life span, the length of time that a female human can conceive—her reproductive period—is also increased. Theoretically, women could continue to ovulate and become pregnant until near death, but unlike men, they do not remain fertile. After about 50 years of age, a woman's ovaries cease to release ova, her monthly menstrual periods stop, and she undergoes menopause. In the latter part of her fertile period, however, the negative effects of 40 years or more of environmental mutagens begin to take their toll. It is advisable for any pregnant woman 35 years or older to have prenatal testing—either amniocentesis or chorionic villus sampling—early in her pregnancy to test for chromosomal abnormalities in her embryo.

From an evolutionary perspective, human menopause is a rather unusual adaptation. If an organism is alive, why should it not be possible for it to reproduce? A human female, with a maximum possible life span of a century, has a reproductive period half that. Human evolution has clearly selected for people to live long postreproductive lives, for reasons probably related to group and kin survival. A family of early hominids with grandmothers must have been a much better bet for survival than one without them. But evolution also limited the tremendous physiological outlay of energy that pregnancy at older ages involves. Older women do not become pregnant because the cost of genetic abnormalities—the "genetic load"—is just too high. Evolution selected for grandmothers to stay alive and well, but for their reproductive capabilities to cease. They pass on their genes vicariously, fostering the survival and successful reproduction of close relatives. This type of evolutionary advantage is known as "inclusive fitness," a topic central to sociobiology, which we discuss in chapter 14.

The evolution of menopause suggests that mutagens have been around in human evolution for a long time. Early on, these mutagens may have been ultraviolet light, dietary toxins, or infectious agents. Today they may be cigarette smoke, drugs, or alcohol. But it is clear that their effects and the resulting evolution at the mother-embryo interface have been important in mammalian evolution. In the evolution of a cessation of ovulation (the remaining several thousand eggs of a woman undergoing menopause are resorbed by the body), natural selection has favored the mother and her kin group over the new individual. At other times when there is a conflict between the interests of the baby and those of the mother, the baby wins. Sometimes, both mother and baby lose. We now turn to this most intimate of evolved human relationships—the nine-month period of time from our conception to birth when we actually live inside another organism, our mother.

The Fetal-Maternal Physiological Bargaining of Pregnancy

All women who have conceived and carried a baby know the major physiological changes wrought by the transformation of pregnancy. The developing embryo first makes the mother give up foods that she previously enjoyed; it then makes her retain fluids, puts an increased demand on her musculoskeletal system, which now must transport a growing amount of weight, alters her sex life by interposing itself between her and her mate, and changes her body form as it grows into a fetus. But the fetus's demands are understandable. It has been compared to an old-style deep-sea diver at depth—entirely dependent on a sustaining lifeline from the surface.

One of the first things that a developing embryo does is establish its own blood supply. The heart starts beating on or about day 21 following conception, the first organ system in the body to become functional. The embryo begins to suck in large amounts of iron, phosphorus, calcium, and protein to make its blood, bones, and muscles. The mother begins to eat voraciously, if she has enough food. Fetal malnutrition occurs at both ends of the socioeconomic scale—the very poor and the wealthy—for very different reasons, but ones which do not matter to the fetus. The affinity that fetal tissues have for calcium and iron is so high that these substances, so important to the mother, will preferentially go to her developing fetus. A poorly nourished pregnant woman may undergo tooth, bone, and hair loss as pregnancy proceeds. There is even a special fat reserve for the fetus that the mother herself cannot use. Female hip and thigh fat is very difficult to reduce by exercise, and it is has been found to be estrogen related in its metabolism. A woman may be close to starvation and may have used up almost all of her subcutaneous fat reserves, but hip and thigh fat will still be conserved, waiting to be called on to sustain the fetus.

The mother's blood volume during pregnancy goes up some 20 percent. If blood volume goes up, so does blood pressure, and if the woman had high blood pressure before, she will potentially have an even greater problem during pregnancy. The fetus is blithely unaware of potential damage to its mother's arteries and kidneys from the hypertension. A good head of pressure is all that more effective in delivering oxygen and nutrients and removing carbon dioxide and wastes. But hypertension of pregnancy, also known as "preeclampsia," is a major health problem for the mother.

Another area of fetal-maternal evolutionary conflict and compromise is the process of birth itself. The head of the human fetus grows faster than that of any other mammal, an indication of the brain's large size. The fetus would likely be happy to stay in the uterus for another month or two because its brain continues to grow at the rapid fetal rate even after birth.[8] But the mother's pelvis, which is only just big enough to accommodate the 40-week-old infant's head, simply couldn't handle anything larger.

A number of evolutionary issues make human birth difficult, both for mother and for baby. First, human bipedality means that the pelvis and the muscles and ligaments of the perineum must support the fetus against the weight of gravity. These structures, particularly the pelvic diaphragm (the "Kegel's muscle" of birth classes), become large and thick, making their stretching around the birth canal during birth slow and painful. In quadrupedal mammals, the pelvic diaphragm is much more lightly constructed because the uterus is supported mainly from the back wall of the pelvis, from which the fetus swings in a fibromuscular hammock.

The human bony pelvis has just about exactly the same inside diameter as the diameter of the head of the fetus. Evolution has not been able to fashion a wider pelvis—humans could not walk and run efficiently with a pelvis any wider than they already have.

So the head of the fetus has evolved to be compressible. Large spaces of unfused skull bones (the "fontanels") allow the head to be molded and squeezed through the birth canal. The pressure exerted on the fetus is tremendous.

A third unique aspect of human birth that makes the process difficult is that the human tail, the coccyx, became flexed under the pelvis, again as part of the pelvic adaptations to bipedality. The fetus's head enters the pelvic cavity upside down and looking to the side, but because the coccyx blocks the way out, its head must turn and flex forward in the birth canal so that it faces either back or front. This twisting of the fetus's body can cause its shoulder to be caught in the birth canal or its neck stretched and injured during birth. Nerve damage causing shoulder droop (Erb-Duchenne palsy) or hand-muscle paralysis ("waiter's tip hand") can result.

The obstetric difficulties that pelvic anatomy and physiology pose has led anthropologist Wenda Trevathan to suggest that human birth is intrinsically a group affair.[9] She maintains that a woman must have assistance in giving birth, and this assistance comes in most cultures from older and experienced women known and trusted by the mother—midwives. How far back in the human evolutionary past midwifery may go is difficult to assess, but it stands to reason that the large cranial size and altered pelvic anatomy of the genus *Homo* may mark the beginnings of a need for it. Anthropologist Mark Skinner has made the suggestion that the well-known Steinheim skull from Germany, a 150,000-year-old *Homo sapiens*, shows the skull asymmetry associated with wryneck. Wryneck, or torticollis, is many times caused by the tearing of one of the large neck muscles in the neck (sternocleidomastoid) when pulling on a baby stuck in the birth canal. The torn muscle later heals but shortens as scar tissue forms, pulling the neck to one side.

Evolution has worked to fashion a closely coordinated physiological communication between mother and baby, clearly of benefit to both. If the birth is successful, the mother passes on her genes, and the baby survives if the mother survives. The modern obstetrician is or should be in the evolutionary role of midwife—an assistance role to the delicately balanced relationship of mother and baby. All too often birth has been considered a medical emergency when it need not be. For example, when women in labor are positioned and immobilized on their backs (the "lithotomy position"), it is a surgical practice inherited from "stonecutters" who removed bladder stones in the days of the barber-surgeons. If a woman is on her back during labor, it makes pushing the baby that much more difficult because she is working against gravity. Women in most cultures squat during birth. These generalizations, however, pertain only to women who are physically prepared for childbirth and do not have some other complicating factor making natural childbirth difficult or impossible. Birth preparation classes can materially assist in the physical challenges of natural childbirth.

Breathing, Bilirubin, and Breast Milk: Entrance into a New World

Once a baby is born, it must make the instant transition that the ancestors of the land vertebrates made over a period of several million years—it must learn to breathe air. There is evidence that the rigors of natural childbirth assist a baby in taking its first breath. The squeezing of the baby's chest during birth expels the amniotic fluid in its lungs, and a cytokine (bradykinin) produced by the baby's body as it is compressed by the uterus begins to close down the channels of blood flow being supplied by the umbilical vein from the placenta to the baby. Babies born by cesarean section may require more assistance in clearing their breathing passages and taking their first breath.

Problems in breathing are the single greatest danger for survival of a premature baby, a fetus expelled too early from its mother's uterus. The lungs were our last major organ system to evolve, and their final development takes place only in the eighth month after conception. If a baby is born too early, it does not have physiologically prepared lungs for breathing. Specifically, it lacks enough "surfactant," a biochemical that creates surface tension on the surfaces of the small air sacs in the lungs and helps them expand. Premature babies need to be coddled in an oxygen-rich environment and kept warm while their lungs mature sufficiently for them to be able to breathe on their own.

Other problems may interfere with a baby's successful breathing. A newborn may be blue not because his or her lungs do not work, but because the mammalian four-chambered heart did not complete its development.[10] Heart defects are among the most common fatal congenital malformations for newborns. Some defects, the so-called left-to-right defects, can be tolerated because oxygenated blood from the left side of the heart leaks over to the right side (with deoxygenated blood returning from the body) and just gets sent redundantly to the lungs. But right-to-left blood shunts in the heart dilute the oxygenated blood returning from the lungs with carbon dioxide–laden blood from the body tissues and recirculates it. Not enough oxygen gets to the tissues, and they turn bluish (the color of deoxygenated blood). Such defects represent a return to the level of an amphibian or even a fish heart, depending on the severity of the malformation. Surgery is usually the only corrective measure for heart defects.

The heart and lungs are not the only immature organs in a human newborn's body. The liver is just getting geared up to produce a number of substances that a free-living organism needs to have. One of these chemicals is glucoronate transferase, an enzyme that attaches an electron to the spent red blood cell protein (bilirubin) to make it water-soluble. This so-called conjugated bilirubin can be excreted in bile through the gallbladder, into the intestine, and finally out of the body in the feces. Some bilirubin also enters the blood from the liver blood supply and is excreted from the blood by the kidney, where it colors the urine yellow. A lot of bilirubin circulating in the blood colors the skin and the whites of the eyes yellow (and the urine a darker yellow), a condition known as jaundice. Newborns do not have enough of the enzyme, so they appear jaundiced a few days after birth. Pediatricians used to be very concerned about this "neonatal jaundice" and prescribed such treatments as bright-light therapy to help the skin metabolize the bilirubin. But if the newborn has a normal liver, evolutionary considerations now make it clear that the relatively high level of bilirubin in a newborn is adaptive.[11] As an oxygen-acceptor molecule, bilirubin acts as a preventive to damage by oxygen free radicals, suddenly in high concentrations, as the newborn's body is flooded with oxygen from the lungs.

High levels of bilirubin also mean high levels of iron in the bloodstream, and bacteria love iron-rich media in which to reproduce. Yet the liver of a newborn also has not yet begun to produce most of the immune system chemicals (immunoglobulins) that are needed for the immune system to fight bacteria. Some immunoglobulins (IgG) made in the mother's body and transferred during pregnancy remain in the newborn's bloodstream after birth, but they are gone after a few days. To counteract bacterial growth and other infections in her newborn, a mother transfers immunoglobulins (IgA) in her breast milk. She also contributes benign bacteria to her suckling infant the same way. The prior presence of benign bacteria prevents the growth of disease-causing bacteria later on. The realization that breast-feeding in a natural (not sterile) environment confers many benefits to a newborn has wrought a slow but profound change on early infant-care practices. Many baby boomers were born in near-sterile hospital conditions and then fed though boiled nipples from bottles filled with sterile, cow milk–based infant formula. Most of us survived, but current practices promise less-severe and less-frequent childhood illnesses, and probably fewer allergic reactions as well.

Diarrheal Disease: The Number One Killer of Babies Worldwide

Diarrhea is the leading cause of infant deaths worldwide. Viral infection (usually a rotavirus), bacterial infection, or parasites account for between 5 and 8 million deaths per year of children under five years of age. Viruses invade the intestines, and the cells then become unable to absorb water and nutrients, producing diarrhea. Bacteria, on the other hand, just preempt the intestinal food resources for their own growth. When they grow too numerous, their waste products (toxins) poison the absorptive intestinal cells. Parasites such as *Giardia* and tapeworms cause diarrhea by damaging cells where they attach to the intestinal walls. Most diarrhea is transmitted by person-to-person (fecal-oral) contact, and it is most common in densely populated areas with inadequate waste treatment facilities and in facilities in which residents lack the knowledge or are incapable of normal personal hygiene. Day-care centers, nursing homes, and refugee camps have high incidences of infectious diarrhea. Death from diarrhea is caused by dehydration, electrolyte (sodium and potassium) imbalance, and malnutrition.

There is evidence that diarrhea has been a killer for thousands of years in human populations. Like malaria, there seems to be a gene mutation that confers some resistance to dehydration from diarrhea. This occurs in the CFTR (cystic fibrosis transmembrane conductance regulator) gene, which, when in single copy, produces a thicker mucus layer in the intestines that serves to conserve water and also absorbs electrolytes across cell membranes (this is why babies with cystic fibrosis can be diagnosed by increased salt levels in their sweat). But again, like malaria, when an individual inherits two copies of the mutated CFTR gene, too much mucus is produced and the disease, cystic fibrosis, clogs the intestines, the lungs, and the pancreas. Cystic fibrosis is the genetic cost of having a genetic change that protects human populations against infectious diarrhea. A CFTR gene mutation is present in 1 in 3,000 Europeans but is less common in other populations, implying that this particular adaptation historically occurred in Europe.

The parameters promoting childhood diarrhea are similar to those of infectious disease in general—high population density and poor sanitation. Neither of these were issues for early hominids because population densities were low and human wastes were easily diluted in the environment. Since at least the Neolithic, humans have become too populous over most of their range to be able to sustain this mode of life. Environmental consciousness and public sanitation have become essential prerequisites of modern life, and they are priorities for the developing nations of the world. To control local outbreaks, hand washing and regular bathing are amazingly effective antidotes.

SIDS and Surviving the Accidents of Infancy and Childhood

Primate infants are not adapted to fending for themselves. All primate mothers, except some human mothers, hold their infants very close to their chests. And in all primates, except humans, the infant can hang on to the convenient body hair of the mother. Human newborns still have this innate clinging ability and will reflexively flex their fingers if their palm is touched. Human newborns are even reputedly able to suspend themselves from a clothesline, but few researchers would admit to trying this.

Anthropologist James McKenna has focused attention on the practice in Western cultures of putting a young infant alone in a bed, perhaps even a more radical thing to do to a primate infant than hanging it from a clothesline.[12] (Recall psychologist Harry Harlow's classic experiments with isolated infant monkeys clinging to even cloth monkey mother surrogates in preference to eating.) Western cultures are virtually unique in separating young infants from their parents at night. The historical practice may have started from a European law in the Renaissance enacted after a baby died when a parent inadvertently smothered him in bed. In the evolutionary past, nighttime would have been the very time when infants would have been held close, to protect them from predation by snakes, leopards, and the like, and perhaps from falling out of the tree. Children's fear of the dark and the monsters that they contain, as well as their proclivity for falling out of bed, are all reflections of this primate evolutionary history.

McKenna has suggested that the practice of separating babies from cosleeping adults is a contributing cause to "sudden infant death syndrome" (SIDS), formerly termed "crib death," for which no clear etiology has yet been determined. McKenna suggests that for a neurologically immature infant, having a parent's heartbeat and warmth close by are important physiological calibrators. If they are not there, the infant may just "forget" to breathe. Other researchers think that asphyxiation from entangling bedclothes, sleeping in a prone position, and smothering from cosleeping adults are greater dangers. The answer is still out on SIDS, but an evolutionary perspective suggests that the species in the primate order and the many non-Western human cultures that practice infant-parent cosleeping cannot be all wrong.

Childhood Allergies, Middle Ear Infections, and Leukemia

Allergy is a recently evolved mammalian response of the immune system to ward off potential mutagens and carcinogens.[13] Specialized immune system cells called mast cells release an immunoglobulin molecule, IgE, newly evolved in mammals, that causes a number of immediate physiological responses.[14] All of these manifestations of allergy are related to expelling irritative substances from the body: sneezing, tear production, coughing, scratching, vomiting, and diarrhea. A drop in blood pressure that accompanies an allergic response helps to slow down the delivery of toxins to the body. Substances that set off an immediate allergic reaction are toxins (mostly from plants) that bind to protein in our blood serum, the nontoxic protein in plants frequently associated with plant toxins, and heavy molecular toxins like bee venom and metals. Authors point out that the aversion of pregnant women to various animal tissues, such as fish or eggs, is explicable. After first exposure, the immune system remembers the substance that first set off the allergic reaction and reacts to it the same way the second time you are exposed to it. Allergies are much more common in industrialized societies than among hunter-gatherers, reflecting a higher exposure to allergenic substances from the environment, mostly pollutants.

When their immune systems become functional, young children are particularly affected by allergies, many of which are airborne. Upper respiratory allergies in children are particularly common, especially in areas where air quality is low, now unfortunately many parts of the developed and developing world. Chronic allergic reactions of the nose and throat, exacerbated by upper respiratory tract viral infections, have caused an epidemic of middle ear infections, due to swelling of the throat lining and blockage of the auditory (eustachian) tubes leading from the throat to the middle ear.[15] Without an open auditory tube, fluid builds up in the middle ear and allows bacterial growth to occur. Pressure, earache, and crying soon follow. Nothing gets a parent's attention more quickly than the latter. Pediatricians prescribe antibiotics to fight the bacterial infection and antihistamines to mute the allergic response in the tissues, but many times these are ineffective measures. An effective surgical solution is a myringotomy (the procedure undertaken to put in "ear tubes") to provide airflow to the middle ear, now the most common surgery on children (following circumcision).[16] Prevention of middle ear infections in children will ultimately be an environmental issue. Adults have much longer auditory tubes than do children, and their allergic responses are usually less severe than those of children, so it may be easier for them to ignore the signs of deteriorating environment and degrading health.

Environmental causes are also paramount in leukemia and other childhood cancers. Leukemia is the most common malignancy among children under the age of 15, and this cancer of the white blood cells is increasing worldwide in its incidence.[17] Exposure of a pregnant woman to carcinogens during pregnancy is the most likely explanation for leukemia afflicting her children after birth. Primary among clearly implicated substances are low-dose radiation, based on a number of studies following the Chernobyl nuclear accident, alcohol use, and diet. An association with paternal cigarette smoking and leukemia in offspring has even been noted. In keeping with our evolutionary understanding of cancer and its cellular causes (chapter 5), we may suspect that any noxious substance that kills cells to which the embryo, or possibly even the sex cells, are exposed may be implicated in causing childhood leukemias and other cancers. Of all the creatures in the environment affected by human polluting, humans themselves will likely suffer the most. The human placenta is the most permeable barrier between the environment and the developing embryo to be found in the animal kingdom. When we pollute our world and poison other species, we can assume that we are also killing ourselves and deforming our children.

4

The Virus War

Modern viruses are relicts of a world so ancient that some deny that it ever existed. Before the first cells, before even DNA, there was an RNA world—naked strings of replicating chemicals called "nucleotides" (Level 1).[1] The discovery of ribozymes (enzymes made of RNA) showed how these proto-organisms fed and reproduced. Today, RNA must use cellular enzymes coded by DNA. And viruses have become parasites, unable to reproduce unless they invade the DNA of cells in other life-forms. They then use the enzymes and the energy sources within the host's cells to produce many more of their own kind.

Viruses cause some of the most dreaded modern diseases, among them AIDS and Ebola hemorrhagic fever. As old as viruses are, they are among the most rapidly evolving of organisms. They are able to evolve to mimic our own cell surface molecules, thus evading detection by our immune defenses. Viruses are sometimes able to jump from one species to another and to insert their genes into our own. Viral zoonoses—animal diseases that spread to humans—result. Viruses can at times hide out in our bodies, quiescent for long periods of time, before erupting into illness.

Medical science has discovered remarkably few drugs that can be used to treat viral infections. None are truly "viricidal," but they can slow down or stop viral reproduction.[2] We may be able to trick our immune systems into recognizing and fighting off viral disease by inoculating ourselves with weakened or dead viruses, such as polio, mumps, measles, or flu. These "attenuated" viruses do not give us the disease, but our immune system will recognize and attack the real thing should it show up. Public health measures, such as eradicating mosquitoes, which spread some viruses, or cleaning public water supplies, have had major beneficial effects on controlling the spread of viral diseases. But our best defense against viruses is still to keep our immune system intact and functioning optimally. This chapter is about human-viral coevolution, how our natural antiviral defenses came into being, and how we can share the planet with viruses without succumbing to them.

The Evolution of Viruses

By most measures, viruses are the most bizarre life-forms still surviving on Earth. They look more like microscopic spacecraft than any sort of organic being. Although we must have shared a common ancestor with viruses, there is precious little to tell us when that might have been. It is possible that an evolutionary split between viruses and all other life-forms was the first evolutionary split in life. It could have happened anytime before about a billion years ago.

A virus has at its core a genetic message encoded in either DNA (deoxyribonucleic acid) or its simpler precursor, RNA (ribonucleic acid). The ribonucleic genome of a virus is quite simple and codes only for the proteins with which the virus coats itself and by which it gains entry into a cell that it is attacking. DNA has a molecular structure with two extra oxygens tacked on, which makes it more stable. RNA is structurally more primitive, and it has fewer enzymes to repair itself. It thus makes more mistakes in replicating itself, but this proneness to genetic mistakes confers on those viruses which use RNA as their molecule of heredity a rapidly changing genetic camouflage. On the other hand, they can stay inert as a virion indefinitely, only reproducing when they come into contact with a cell to invade. Viruses do not have to replicate at all to stay "alive."

The anatomy of a virus is also simple. An encircling covering, a capsid, surrounds and protects its fragile genetic molecule. In most viruses an envelope surrounds the capsid. The envelope has neuraminidase (NA) molecules over about 20 percent of its surface, with which it dissolves the cell membranes of prey cells. It has hemagglutinin (HA) molecules over the remaining 80 percent of its surface, which it uses to dock with and attach to cells it will invade. The HA molecules of a virus are ever changing because of its rapidly evolving genome, rendering it a moving target for our immune system to recognize. This is the reason that every fall, if you are exposed to the flu, you will either get it (your immune system will not recognize the new viral strain and fail to attack it) or you will need to get a flu shot (so that you will develop antibodies to an attenuated infusion of the virus). There will have been enough evolution in the influenza A virus over a year's time that your body will no longer recognize the new strain, even if you had the flu the preceding season.

Although the ways of viruses are many and varied, many seem to have a proclivity for animal blood. Their ancient adaptation may have been to invade blood cells, reproduce, and then cause the host's body to hemorrhage them and their progeny out again into the environment. Three distantly related viral families (filoviruses, arenaviruses, and flaviviruses) cause hemorrhagic disease, suggesting that this adaptation may be primitive for the entire group. Viruses need water to live and spread. If they dry out, they die. Any way that fluids pass between organisms—droplets from a sneeze, blood from a mosquito or tick bite, shaking hands and then touching the edge of the eye, exchange of sexual fluids, or by injections from unsterile needles—can potentially transmit viruses.

Virus Ecology: Zoonoses and Vectors

The most horrifying viruses come out of the tropical forests, especially the forests of Africa: HIV, Ebola, West Nile, and yellow fever, to name a few. Africa is, after all, where most of the last 40 million years of our evolution has taken place, and it makes sense that many viruses have coevolved to parasitize African primates, including ourselves. We may have spread beyond the African forests starting 2.5 million years ago, but we remain susceptible to their viruses.

Viruses, as relics of a watery RNA world, proliferate where water is abundant. On land, these habitats tend to be forests. Leaving a number of viral infections behind in the forest may not have been an entirely coincidental benefit of hominid colonization of the savanna. Chimps, gorillas, and our more distant relatives, the monkeys and the prosimians, have served to keep African forest primate viruses alive, well, and evolving. They can jump species boundaries when given a chance.

The health threat of African viruses is real, but our fear is exacerbated by their novelty. We live with many more common viruses that can vault over species barriers much closer to home. Molecular analyses show, surprisingly, that many viruses that infect modern humans date from only the last 7,000 to 8,000 years.[3] Considering the antiquity of viruses and their parasitic relationship with higher organisms, the recency of this date requires some explanation. It comes not only from viruses' ability to evolve rapidly, but also opportunity—the unusual evolutionary event of humans bringing into close biological proximity entire animal populations that were previously separate and distinct from the standpoint of their viruses.

Animal domestication dates from the last 10,000 years or so. The close association of human and nonhuman species offers tremendous advantages to viruses. They have different animal population reservoirs in which to evolve and build up antigenic differences, and then easy infection routes when they reinfect humans. These common human viruses are largely non-African in origin. The influenza virus likely arose in birds and possibly spread to humans from Asian jungle fowls, the first domesticated ancestors of the chicken. Pigs, domesticated from European wild boars, also harbor the influenza virus and are additional candidates for where the disease originated. The smallpox virus shares a reservoir with cows. Other viruses are shared with sheep, rodents, carnivores, and other species.

Viruses, we must remember, are organisms with very limited capabilities. Active movement is one ecological adaptation they lack. They may be in close proximity to a population of potential hosts, but they must have a ride into their wet cellular interiors in order to infect and reproduce. Sometimes we help the viruses, as when we appose wet surfaces on our bodies—for example, in kissing, which can spread Epstein-Barr virus (the cause of mononucleosis and Burkitt's lymphoma), or in sex, which can spread herpes and the HIV virus. But many other viruses require other mechanisms to get into our bodies. These are called "vectors."

Some animal species coevolving with viruses have become very effective vectors of human viral diseases. In general, any species that can pierce human skin is an excellent candidate for a virus to use to infect a human host. Ticks and fleas have strong mandibles with which they can bite through human skin to feed on blood. Viruses use this adaptation as their insect vector to make the jump from whatever species the flea or tick last bit to a human. Haired mammals that sleep in the same place for at least two weeks (the average length of the tick and flea life cycle) are favorite hosts. The argument has been made that avoiding this type of parasitism was a major evolutionary advantage of human hairlessness, especially after early humans began living in semipermanent home bases (Level 16).

The major insect agent transmitting viruses to humans, however, is the mosquito. Dozens of viral diseases, the most famous being yellow fever, enter the human body, and travel between humans, via the proboscis of these bloodsucking insects. This mechanism of viral injection is so effective that other types of pathogens, such as the malarial parasite, have also evolved to utilize it.

Just as you can prevent rabies by avoiding being bitten by a rabid dog, so can you prevent many insect-borne diseases by avoiding or counteracting mosquito bites. Mosquito repellent, screens over your windows, mosquito nets around your bed, clothing that protects your neck, arms, and legs, and living away from mosquito breeding areas with standing water are all effective preventive strategies. We also have some anatomical defenses. The small hairs covering most parts of our bodies, a vestige of our dense apelike mantle of hair, may well serve to detect insects landing. The widespread Western practice of women shaving their legs accounts for their generally receiving many more mosquito bites than men. The greater thickness of Africans' skin, compared to other, hairier human populations, may also be an adaptation to withstanding the attacks of pathogen-bearing biting insects in the tropics.

Despite our first lines of defense, viruses may, and eventually will, succeed in gaining entrance to our body. We have a complex of evolved internal defenses that effectively help us in warding off viral diseases.

The Evolution of Viral Defenses: The Immune System

In the beginning, viruses may have preyed on beings very much like themselves—naked ribonucleic acid molecules floating around in the primeval seas—but they later specialized on getting into the DNA of bacteria-like prokaryotes. They still attack bacteria today. Single-celled prokaryotes have DNA organized into densely packed chromosomes that they protect inside a cell membrane. Using neuraminidase like a burglar's acetylene torch, a virus rappels down the cell wall with a hemagglutinin receptor molecule, dissolves a hole in the bacterial cell membrane, and then ducks inside. It traverses the dangerous territory between the cell wall and the chromosome, its goal, as quickly as possible, in order to avoid the prokaryote's internal defenses. The prokaryote may produce a poisonous substance, such as the cholera toxin released by the bacterium *Vibrio cholerae* when it is invaded by a virus. Similar defenses that arose in our single-celled ancestors signaled the beginning of our immune system.

As soon as one of our cells picks up the telltale sign of a viral intruder—double-stranded RNA (made by both RNA and DNA viruses)—it immediately begins to make interferon. Every cell in the human body still has this ability. Interferon is a protein that stimulates the production of an enzyme called RNase, which degrades single-stranded RNA, thus inactivating the virus. Interferon also heads off the virus's attempt at taking over the cell's genetic machinery by shutting down its own protein-making activity (translation of the DNA message into protein). And interferon can also stimulate the production of so-called Mx proteins, which prevent the replication of some viruses.

Higher organisms, like plants and animals, evolved an additional inner perimeter of defense against viral invasion by forming a membrane around their chromosomes. This inner sanctum became the nucleus of the eukaryote ("true chromosome") cell. It also made possible separate chemical reactions in the nucleus and in the outer fluid space, the cytoplasm, of the cell. As we saw in chapter 2, the first eukaryote cell ancestors formed a coevolutionary pact with other primitive prokaryote cells that came into the cytoplasm for protection. In return, the harboring cells specialized for certain functions. One such function was fighting off cell invaders. It made good sense to reuse the proteins and chemical elements in invaders into the cell, so one approach was just to eat them. Lysosomes are cell organelles descended from ancient prokaryotes that specialized for this function. Peroxisomes evolved to kill invading viruses and bacteria by hitting them with a blast of hydrogen peroxide.

With the appearance of multicellular organisms, defense, like most other functions, was largely taken over by specialized cells. Cell-mediated immunity had evolved by the time of the first animals (Level 5). Natural killer cells roamed the early circulatory system in search of strange or unknown intruders. They identified them by the presence of molecules called "opsonins" that attached themselves to foreign substances in the body. This process of opsonization was the first step in defining what a multicellular organism considered "self" and "non-self." Everything falling into the latter category was attacked and degraded. Today, this system still functions in our body and is called the "complement" system, so named because it assists the immune system in identifying and neutralizing pathogens.

Over time attackers became more sophisticated. Like the ancient Greeks who penetrated the city walls of Troy by hiding inside a wooden horse, viruses, bacteria, and parasites cloaked themselves in proteins that could evade the complement system. The immune system responded by evolving more sophisticated means of identifying non-self invaders. An organ, the thymus, which evolved in the lower neck region, served as a nursery for developing immune cells. "T cells" (named after the thymus) were educated here as to the surface chemical characteristics of the body's cells. These surface characteristics are determined by genes in the major histocompatibility complex (MHC). T cells attack any cells that they find within the body that do not pass the test of familiar MHC patterns. To further speed up the body's response to invasion, "memory B" cells evolved that could "remember" the cell surface characteristics of past invaders or infections. Memory B cells produce "antibodies," chemicals that tangle up and degrade any pathogens that attempt to invade the body again. The immune system is effective in detecting and eliminating the rapidly changing viral and bacterial pathogens that attempt to infect it, but it is a constant evolutionary battle.

The Spread of Viruses

Within only the past few thousand years, a number of viral diseases have appeared. Their toll in human suffering and mortality has been significant. The time frame in which they have emerged suggests that they are diseases of civilization—evolved in response to quite recent changes in human evolution (Level 17). Many may be prevented or preventable.

Viruses, as a group, are well adapted to infect human beings. Both viruses and humans move fast. When humans move into a new area, begin new activities, and begin doing old activities in different ways, viruses are there, ready to evolve and take advantage of the new conditions. The waning years of the Ice Age, beginning after 18,000 years ago, was a period of great virus expansion as virions woke up out of a long deep freeze. When humans domesticated animals—first the dog, then the goat, the horse, the cow, the pig, the chicken, and other species—beginning after about 10,000 years ago, viruses gained tremendous opportunities for interspecies spread. And when people started living in larger population centers called villages at about the same time, viral populations expanded accordingly.

The most famous virus of our time, HIV, is a good example of how readily a recently emerging virus can spread.[4] Originally a denizen of the ancient central African forests, HIV was roused out of its normal chimpanzee host species by any one of several human activities—chimp hunters getting the virus through infected blood on their hands, a human having been bitten by an infected chimp, or even infected chimp liver cells being used to culture polio vaccines in central Africa in the late 1950s. Except for very small numbers of "pygmy" tribes like the Mbuti, hominids had not ventured into the dense rain forests of Africa since the Miocene. As people encroach on these environments, which host wet-loving viruses adapted to infecting our close primate relatives, more previously quiescent viruses will turn up, and we will be subjected to more mysterious infections. As human population continues to increase and as people increasingly move about the globe, new viruses or new strains of old viruses will spread with them. We know that AIDS spread along the Trans-Africa Highway extending east and west out of the forests of the eastern Congo, and down the Zaire River. These routes led to large population centers like Nairobi and Kinshasa, and with their busy international airports, it was only a question of time before opportunistic HIV viruses made the trip out of Africa.

Population centers and airports have a lot to do with the spread of other human viruses. With a constant supply of immunologically naive hosts to infect and a worldwide transportation network to reach them, viruses can flourish.

Influenza—the "flu"—which infects hundreds of millions of people annually, is probably the most widely spread disease in the world. Many of us in the United States contract it each year, and flu accounts for countless sick days lost from work and school. The 1918 influenza pandemic following World War I accounted for 25 million deaths worldwide, and its virulence is still unexplained.[5] This seems like an onerous burden of disease from an evolutionary standpoint, and it is.

The virus that causes influenza is classified as an orthomyxovirus, discovered in 1933. The disease, however, has been recognized since at least the 18th century, when Italians considered bad air and inauspicious astrological signs to be responsible for disease-causing "influences." The flu virus, however, is spread by moist droplets expelled from the nose or mouth in a sneeze or a cough. Like many pathogens, the flu virus's symptoms in a human host facilitate the dissemination and spread of the virus. The virus strikes with greatest force when the immune response is decreased, in concert with fatigue, stress, and other illness. It is not usually fatal, although it may make human patients so miserable that they may think that they are going to die. When you get the flu and recover, your antibodies protect you from another infection, and you are unlikely to contract it again in the same flu season. But when another year rolls around, you get the flu again. There has been enough evolution in the new flu virus strain to outdistance the immune system's recognition of last year's virus. A number of considerations argue against this state of affairs being a stable evolutionary situation.

How do you fight back against the flu? First off, banish the thought that modern medicine is going to vanquish the flu virus. It will be here far longer than our species. But there are tried-and-true methods to use to avoid the flu. You can keep viruses away by creating a dry, virus-free buffer zone around yourself, since flu viruses, like all viruses, have to have water to live and spread. Your palms are always somewhat moist and harbor viruses, so frequent hand washing is a simple but extremely effective way to avoid the flu. Droplets also transmit flu viruses, and keeping other people from sneezing on you, or near you, is important in avoiding infection.

Our species also has an evolutionarily old and effective defense against viral attack, and it is important to keep your immune system in good shape. If you are run down and stressed, your immune system cannot adequately fight off a viral invasion should one occur. If you want to give your immune system a boost, a flu shot with the attenuated version of the most recent strain of the flu virus is a good way to do it. You are merely reproducing the close coevolutionary relationship between your immune system and the flu virus that has existed for millennia. Our skin is our main defense against viruses because it is generally dry, impermeable to water and blood, and sealed off from the environment. Most viruses enter our body from a defect in the skin or mucous linings, made either by the agent causing the infection, such as a mosquito, or incidental to the viral invasion. Keeping our skin intact is perhaps an obvious, but still very important, step in preventing viral disease.

Coevolution and Autoimmune Disease

Sometimes, and not all that infrequently, the virus wins in its ecological competition with us. Luckily, this does not mean that we
die. The virus can gain its evolutionary objectives—to reproduce—
and we can continue to gain ours—to reproduce. In fact, the virus's
evolutionary strategy is more successful if it propagates many
copies of itself, and if it can do this by a less virulent and less
aggressive approach than killing off its host, then natural selection
will favor that adaptation.

Some viruses become adept at hiding out in our body, adopting
a biochemical camouflage that evades detection by the immune
system. They evolve surface proteins that mimic those of certain of
our body cells so closely that white blood cells and macrophages
simply pass them by. The viruses wait until the time is right, perhaps when the immune system is weakened or occupied with fighting another infection, and then they reproduce. As they infect
more cells, the immune system detects the signs of cellular damage
and hones in on the virally infected cells. But when the immune
system finds the antigen, it seems to be the body's own cells. B cells
nevertheless make an antibody to it. Now our body has begun to
attack itself, and the virus has won the battle of immunological
mimicry. The diseases thus caused are termed "autoimmune diseases."

For the lurking virus's wait-and-see strategy to work, it needs to
infect a cell type that is long lived. Nerve cells, which are not con-
stantly replaced in the body like most other cells, are perfect targets. Most recognized autoimmune diseases indeed affect nerve
cells or cells in specific organs that develop from nerve cells. One
example is insulin-dependent diabetes mellitus, also called
juvenile-onset or type I diabetes (to be distinguished from type II,
adult-onset, non-insulin-dependent diabetes, discussed in chapter
9). Autoantibodies attack specific insulin-secreting cells in the
pancreas, beta cells in the islet of Langerhans, destroying them.
These cells develop from embryonic gut tissue in association with
neural crest (amine precursor uptake and decarboxylation, or
APUD) cells migrating in from the embryonic nervous system to
form the future glandular tissue of the pancreas. A viral infection
preceding the onset of type I diabetes is common, but not always

diagnosed or observed. Associations have been observed between infections of mumps, hepatitis, mononucleosis, rubella ("German measles"), Coxsackie, and other viral infections. Current evidence, although not yet conclusive, even suggests that a virus causes type I diabetes.[6] Table 4 lists other common autoimmune diseases that are generally accepted to be caused by similar viral subterfuge.

Causing autoimmune disease is not really the virus's goal when it infects a human host. Its evolutionary strategy is merely to avoid detection by a cloaking maneuver—wrapping itself and the cell it infects with an immunologically invisible covering. The cell infected does not have to be a nervous-system-derived cell, but these cells do seem among the most common viral targets. The AIDS virus, on the other hand, uses a different strategy—undermining the entire immune system to avoid detection and attack. This latter adaptation is a more recently evolved endgame, and it can result in the relatively rapid death of the host (usually not advantageous from the virus's perspective). We could expect that a virus like HIV might evolve to be less fatal over time, and this indeed may be one reason that HIV has not accounted for as high a mortality rate among AIDS patients as first feared.

Autoimmune diseases are still poorly understood and difficult for physicians to treat. Because there are few if any effective antiviral drugs for any specific infection, doctors treat the symptoms of

Table 4. Some Common Autoimmune Diseases

Pancreas:	*Thyroid:*
Type I diabetes mellitus	Graves' disease, Hashimoto's thyroiditis
Suprarenal:	*Neuromuscular System:*
Autoimmune Addison's disease	Multiple sclerosis, myasthenia gravis, Guillain-Barré syndrome
Connective Tissue:	*Vasculature:*
Rheumatoid arthritis, systemic lupus erythematosus, psoriasis, Sjögren's syndrome	Takayasu's arteritis, Kawasaki's disease, temporal arteritis, Wegener's granulomatosis

Adapted from Fauci, A. S. et al., eds. 1998. *Harrison's Principles of Internal Medicine,* 14th ed. New York: McGraw-Hill.

the disease. Drugs to suppress the immune system or inflammation, such as steroids, are sometimes prescribed, but overuse opens the door to other infections and negative side effects. If a viral infection or autoimmune reaction causes cellular destruction, as is the case in type I diabetes mellitus, the product of the destroyed cells—insulin—can be replaced by injection. Only clearer understanding of the evolution and exact causation of the various viral diseases will eventually lead to better treatment and prevention. For example, the Ebola virus is still harbored by an unknown forest- or perhaps cave-living organism in one of the ancient forest refuges of Africa. Until we find out where it hides between its periodic virulent outbreaks in humans, it will be impossible to adequately prevent its depredations.

It is likely that we and our chromosome-bearing ancestors have shared Earth with viruses for well over a billion years. Juxtaposed to this immense span of time, it is clear that human viral infections have increased in frequency since the last ice age, and especially since the domestication of animals. The increases in viral and related autoimmune diseases in the last century have been related to greater contact with viral reservoirs in animal populations, higher human population density, and increasing population movements as international travel and development have increased. These trends show no sign of diminishing in the future. Our best chances of preventing viral diseases lie with avoiding the vectors that spread viruses and keeping our immune systems strong.

5

Cellular Stress: A General Model for Cancer

Modern medicine, congratulating itself for the near-successful eradication of infectious disease during the latter part of the 20th century, turned its attention to finding a cure for cancer. Cancer is an uncontrolled proliferation of cells that forms tumors—masses that can grow, spread, then seed new tumors in distant sites around the body. By the end of the millennium a cure had still not been found, although today an estimated one-third of all people in the industrialized world will develop some form of cancer.[1] Indeed, some years ago the largely runaway rate of cancer was called the "failure of medicine."[2] Certainly, compared to the conquering of virtually all infectious diseases in the industrialized world, our powerlessness in the face of cancer is striking.

Is medicine still on the right track, or is something wrong with the paradigm that medical scientists are using to search for a cure? Can we do anything on our own to prevent cancer? If we are diagnosed with a type of cancer, is there anything we can do to alleviate its effects? To answer these questions, we will review what medicine knows about cancer and then interpret this knowledge in light of our evolutionary biology.

Of Tumors and Rudolf Virchow

In 1855 an eminent German pathologist and anthropologist, Rudolf Virchow of Berlin, first proposed that cancer arose not from congealed body fluids or vaguely defined fibers, but from other cells. This opinion reversed speculations on the causes of cancer going back to antiquity—to Hippocrates and the ancient Egyptians. Virchow and legions of successive generations of pathologists have chronicled the microscopic changes that cells undergo when they become cancerous. Still today, in operating theaters around the world, all surgery stops while a microscopic determination by a pathologist is made to determine if a bit of cellular tissue removed from a patient is cancerous. This cellular perspective has been very effective in diagnosing cancer when it occurs, but that is often too late for the patient. The origins of cancer need to be understood so that the disease can be cut off much earlier, even before it starts.

Medicine has pinned much of its hopes for finding a cure for cancer on genetics, and genes do play an important role in the development of cancerous cells, just as they do in the development and ongoing functions of all cells in our bodies. So in the sense that genes are in the chain of development of cancer, they can be said "to cause cancer," but they do not lie at the very root of the problem. The breakdown is in the cooperation between cells.

Thus, medicine's approach to understanding cancer cannot be focused only on single cells, but at a higher level of organization—on the whole organism. Cancer is a Level 4 rather than a Level 3 disease. Phrased in evolutionary terms, single-celled organisms cannot have cancer. They may just divide more rapidly or in a disorganized manner. The disease is by definition one that affects multicellular organisms—when some cells rebel against the system. Virchow and succeeding pathologists were so focused on the cell theory, looking at single cells (which did serve to document cancer when it occurred), that they overlooked that fact that cancer is a phenomenon of cells in groups. And the cells interact among themselves and with the environment. Cancer is only understandable as an ecological disease.

Ecology is ironically the science founded by Virchow's arch-rival, Ernst Haeckel, Germany's foremost Darwinian. Haeckel realized that the adaptations of organisms evolved in intimate connection with their environments. But Virchow and his contemporaries, not having knowledge of either the mechanisms responsible (genetics) or the historical documents of evolution (fossils), considered that evolutionary biology was too speculative.

Virchow did eventually acknowledge, however, that the environment was the prime mover in cancer. In 1893 he hypothesized that environmental irritants caused cancerous growths. Still focusing on the cell itself, though, he said that "the cell possesses the characteristic of irritability, and changes in its substance, provided they do not destroy life, produce disease."[3] As soon as he invoked the environment as the probable cause of cancer, Virchow left the domain of the single cell and entered into the preserve of ecology and the whole organism. Today, Virchow's fundamental principles of pathology make eminent sense in light of evolutionary biology. His famous exhortation that "pathological formations never develop beyond the physiological possibilities of the species"[4] can in fact form the starting point for our evolutionary hypothesis of cancer.

A New Paradigm for Cancer

Animal species in the wild have not been observed to contract cancer. Animals only get cancer when they live in captivity for many years or are subjected to medical experiments intended to generate cancerous tumors. Nonindustrialized peoples do not contract cancer. What is it about living in the industrialized world that gives animals, including us, cancer?

Recent research and an evolutionary perspective suggest that stress on our cells and their response to that stress underlie most cancers. To understand cancer, let us regress to the Archean era, a billion years ago. Single-celled organisms such as bacteria are the highest life-forms, and they fend for themselves. If a bacterium experiences too much heat, too much cold, too much radiation, not enough food, crowding with other bacteria, poisons, or invasion by other life-forms, it reacts. Initially, it may produce one of a wide variety of protective proteins, such as the so-called heat shock proteins. If a virus enters it, a cell may produce an oxidative burst, attacking the invaders with hydrogen peroxide or caustic nitrite bleach.

When cells began to live together and cooperate inside whole organisms, composed of many different cells types, the original single cells employed one of their primitive adaptations to stop growing. When they became crowded, they slowed down their metabolism and stopped dividing. Many small genetic adaptations occurred over evolutionary time that fine-tuned this adaptation as cells mutually adopted a pact of cooperativity. Cancer is a breakdown of this pact between cells within an organism.

The dual nature of cells—their self-centered individual functions and their contributions to the organism-centered body as a whole—was noted by one of the discoverers of cells, Matthias Schleiden, in the early 19th century. Cells that turn cancerous lose their organism-centered identity and become wholly self-centered.

If bacteria that have been hemmed in by other bacteria suddenly sense that their neighbors are no longer there, they immediately begin to divide and grow. A similar primitive cellular mechanism underlies cancer. A cell in the body senses that cells around it are dying or dead and its ancient cellular machinery kicks into gear, causing it to undergo rapid self-replication as if it were once again a free-living cell. The key event here is the nearby injury or death of cells that trigger the initial carcinogenic process. Once that process starts, it is difficult to stop, and it will usually continue until the rogue cells that have rebelled against the pact of cooperativity in the body are killed.

Two sorts of genes drive this process. Those that promote rapid cell division and growth are termed "oncogenes" ("onco-" is from the Latin for "tumor"). They turn on after some insult to the cell—an "irritant" in Virchow's terminology. These are the messages that tell an individual cell to divide as rapidly as possible because it is all alone and must act quickly to keep its gene line alive. Then there are "tumor suppressor genes." These are genes that put a brake on cell division. They evolved in social archaeobacteria that grew in colonies and had to have some way to stop dividing when they met bacteria of their own ilk.

If this model for cancer is correct, why do cancerous cells keep on growing? Why, when they reach other cells clearly organized as functioning tissue, do they aggressively grow into them, disrupting them? Consider the situation from the cell's point of view. Assaulted on all sides by noxious substances or foreign agents, it may consider its compact with its neighboring cells null and void. As a result, when a growing group of cancerous cells reaches normal tissue, they no longer recognizes it as "self." To the cancerous cells, normal tissue within the body might as well be a piece of primeval sea rock which the cancer can colonize. The tumor will only stop when it reaches cells of its own kind—in this case, other cancerous cells. By this point, cancerous cells have metastasized all over the body, and the organism is dead.

In the long-ago Archean era, this behavior of single-celled organisms living in colonies would have been adaptive. After an environmental disruption severe enough to kill off neighboring cells, natural selection would favor surviving cells that reproduced rapidly and expanded into the available space around themselves. The surviving cells would not know why they survived. Was it that they were slightly more impervious to the ultraviolet radiation, more resistant to raised temperatures, had better repair mechanisms for damaged DNA, or maybe were just lucky? It did not matter. There was space available, and they reproduced. Modern cells retain this capability. Cancer in this view, then, is not a collapse of cellular function, but rather an inappropriate activation of an ancient adaptive mechanism. In Virchow's terminology, cancer turns out to be, like other pathology, within the "physiological possibilities of the species."

Given that this primitive adaptation of cells is so old and so maladaptive to modern people, why did natural selection not remove it? The answer lies in how evolution works. Adaptations evolve from prior adaptations, not as de novo innovations. Our earliest colonial-living, single-celled ancestors were "proto-organisms" in the sense that they all had only one type of cell. There was no division of labor among the cells. Great mats of algal stromatolites living today along the Great Barrier Reef in Australia are a good analogue of this very early stage of our evolution. When certain types of cells in one part of the colony evolved to do some things that other cells did not, the colony became transformed into an organism—a multicelled being with cell types that cooperate. For example, cells at one end of the organism developed waving little arms called "cilia" that wafted currents and nutrients into the organism. Others on the outside of the organism developed thicker cell membranes for protection. Cells along the sides of the organism developed the ability to change shape and contract, thus allowing movement of the organism. Over immense spans of time—well over a billion years— evolution by natural selection produced organisms whose cooperating cellular components survived better than did unspecialized cells living in colonies. But in the new organisms, the intrinsic nature of the cells did not change. The cells just added new capabilities. These capabilities provided some benefit to the other cells living within the organism, but they also made possible benefits from those other cells as well. We retain today, for better or for worse, the heritage of our earliest single-celled ancestors. Cancer also seems to be a recent disease, and one that affects people later in life, after they have reproduced. Natural selection has not had enough time or acted with sufficient force to significantly reduce the incidence of cancer under the environmental conditions in which we live.

Creating Cancer

Many researchers have searched for decades for specific chemical or biological agents that are associated with particular cancers. There are many, but they all share one characteristic. They, or the concentrations in which they enter the body, are evolutionarily novel. Our body's evolved immune, detoxifying, and excretionary systems are just not up to the task of handling these substances because this sort of stress is new to human evolution. Natural selection is now responding by exacting a toll in human mortality and morbidity that in turn will affect the gene pool of successive generations. Those individuals with a tolerance for the environmental toxins and other carcinogenic agents of the modern world, or on whom the effects are delayed far past reproductive age, will be favored by natural selection. To effect major change, however, future evolution will have to continue for several tens of thousands of years. For those of us who may want to work within our current biological limits, there is another possible solution—identify the carcinogens and reduce their concentrations.

Table 5 sets out a list of the some of the known major human carcinogens. Several caveats are necessary before interpreting this table. First, laboratory experiments have amply demonstrated that almost any substance in high-enough concentration in the living environment of an organism is potentially carcinogenic. So the concept here is not that only certain substances are harmful and can cause cancer, but that all biologically active substances in our environment should be maintained within certain limits—those limits established by the ancestral environments to which we are adapted. Second, the exact degree of carcinogenicity for many substances in humans is difficult to determine because (a) animal species on which the substance may have been tested are not humans and do not share all or even many aspects of our biology, (b) human beings generally live a long time, and carcinogens may exert their effects years later, and (c) we are affected by many substances and potential carcinogenic agents simultaneously, thus making it difficult or impossible to determine which one factor, if only one, may be the most important in causing cancer. Many researchers think in fact that there is a "dosage effect" of many carcinogens, each individually below the threshold of cancer but collectively carcinogenic.

There are several general categories of carcinogens. Poisons, such as hydrocarbons, directly damage cells. Sir Percival Pott first discovered this link in his classic study of chimney sweeps in 18th-century London. Soot inside their clothes caused cancer of the scrotum. In this case prevention was simple: sweeps needed a daily bath. Indeed, a recent study of Swedish chimney sweeps, who now take regular baths, showed no increase in scrotal cancer compared to the general population. Hydrocarbons are also one of the primary carcinogenic agents in cigarette smoke, to be discussed in chapter 8.

Hormones can also be carcinogenic. Evolved to be "exciting" and powerful communicating substances, they promote the growth of cells with the appropriate receptors on their surfaces. Too much of them can cause cancer in the tissues they target. For example, an

Table 5. A Partial List of Carcinogenic Substances and Processes

Aflatoxins
Aluminum production
4-aminobiphenyl
Analgesic mixtures containing phenacetin
Arsenic and arsenic compounds
Asbestos
Auramine manufacture
Azathioprine
Benzene
Benzidine
Betel quid with tobacco
Bis(chloromethyl) ether and chloromethyl methyl ether (technical grade)
Boot and shoe manufacture and repair
1,4-butanediol dimethanesulfonate (Myleran)
Chlorambucil
Chromium compounds, hexavalent
Coal gasification
Coal tar pitches
Coal tars
Coke production
Diethylstilbestrol
Estrogen replacement therapy
Estrogen, nonsteroidal
Estrogen, steroidal
Furniture and cabinet working
Hematite mining, underground, with exposure to radon
Iron and steel founding
Isopropyl alcohol manufacture, strong-acid process
Magenta manufacture
Melphalan
8-Methoxypsoralen (Methoxsalen) plus ultraviolet radiation
Mineral oils, untreated and mildly treated
Mustard gas (sulfur mustard)
2-naphthylamine
Nickel and nickel compounds
Oral contraceptives, combined
Oral contraceptives, sequential
Rubber industry
Shale oils
Soots
Talc-containing asbestiform fibers
Tobacco products, smokeless
Tobacco smoke
Vinyl chloride

Adapted from Harrison's Internal Medicine Online 2001, Table 390-2.

imbalance of male hormones, or androgens, is implicated in prostate cancer. Excess female hormones, or estrogens, taken as old-style birth control pills (diethylstilbestrol) or increased in a woman over the years because of delayed pregnancy, can stimulate cancers of the reproductive system and probably breast cancers, to be discussed in chapter 6.

Viruses can cause cancer. For example, the Epstein-Barr virus causes Burkitt's lymphoma, and the human papillomavirus causes cervical cancer. Viruses were undoubtedly ancient competitors of our single-celled ancestors, and their attacks did not cease when our cells became communally organized into organisms. Viruses invade cells' DNA and co-opt the cellular machinery to reproduce themselves. Rapid cellular replication can be a way viruses manipulate the cell to produce more of their kind, or it can be yet another cellular response to injury. The association of Kaposi's sarcoma and the HIV virus is only one well-known example.

Bacteria and parasites are more recent enemies of our cells, and they are also implicated in certain cancers. Some of the earliest known cancerous tumors, found in Egyptian mummies, are bladder tumors likely caused by schistosome parasites endemic to the Nile River.

Any medical conditions or substances that decrease our body's resistance and impair immune functions increase cellular injury and thus increase the chances of cancer. Immunosuppressive agents used in patients with organ transplants, for example, have been implicated in non-Hodgkin's lymphoma, a suite of cancers of the white blood cells.

The multifarious causes of cancer are confusing until one realizes their underlying similarity. They all cause cellular injury. And cells react to that injury in an evolutionarily predictable way—by proliferating. That response is no longer adaptive, but its origin can now be explained. Modern research on the genetics of cancer is adding detail to the story.

Cancer as a Disease of DNA

Genetic research in recent years has demonstrated the mechanism by which cells are turned into replicating machines, as they abdicate their organismal responsibilities and begin to act like primitive single cells again. Specific types of genes called regulatory genes determine when and how fast a cell replicates. Genes that turn on or speed up replication have been marketed (for the cancer-research funding organizations) as "proto-oncogenes." They really do not have anything specifically to do with cancer ("onco-") when they are functioning normally. There are also regulatory genes that slow down or stop cell replication. These have been termed tumor suppressor genes. We can simply call them "go genes" and "stop genes."

When go genes are mutated by carcinogens, they get turned on all the time, making their proteins continuously and causing cells to enter the replication phase of their life cycle. As soon as this happens, the go gene becomes a cancer-causing gene. Stop genes, on the other hand, work normally by causing a cell to die a natural death ("apoptosis" in medical terminology) when it becomes old or unneeded. They also may mutate, ceasing their euthanasic function, and the cancerous cells may become "immortal," at least for a while.

What is interesting about the genetics of cancer is that the same mutations consistently appear in specific cancers and occur at the same specific points on the chromosomes (which are therefore called "point mutations"). Lung cancer masses, for example, have *ras* gene mutations in their cells (*ras*, the best-known sarcoma, is short for "rat sarcoma" because it was first found in lab rodents). The point mutations are in specific places (codons 12 or 61) and disrupt the "G-protein" turnoff switch for the gene. Cancerous tumors in the bladder, the colon, and the pancreas also are characterized by ras gene mutations.

There is clearly a pattern here. When conditions in the cell's environment become intolerable, and neighboring cells begin dying, with perhaps even damage to the cell itself, go and stop genes mutate out of their cooperative states and go into a self-centered survival mode. There is every indication that this reaction is an evolved adaptation, and that it is ancient.

Two other genetic changes that have been observed in cancerous cells have the same effect—they allow the injured cells to replicate rapidly. When pressed by carcinogenic forces, a cell's DNA can act to duplicate portions that contain oncogenes, thus increasing their effects on cell replication. Cellular pathologists see such amplified DNA in cancerous cells in the form of tiny iso-lated chromosomal fragments, termed "double minutes" (because they are formed from each chromosome in a pair and because they are minute). Sometimes such amplified sections stay integrated into whole chromosomes. But the effect is the same. Oncogenes contained within the section of amplified DNA are increased in number and accelerate cell growth. In breast cancer, for example, the *erbB2* oncogene is amplified within double minutes found in cancerous breast tissue.

A related type of genetic mutation associated with cancer is the breaking of chromosomes at go gene sites, associated with greater production of molecules that promote cell replication. Bro-ken chromosomes have sticky ends and can rearrange themselves. Such translocations of broken pieces of chromosomes are seen in a number of cancers. Burkitt's lymphoma, for example, a disease of white blood cells, has characteristic translocations between chro-mosomes 8 and 14. The result of such chromosomal rearrange-ments is to increase replication of the affected cells without regard to messages from other cells in the body—cancer.

Could cancer ever be adaptive to an organism? The answer is almost certainly no. Cancer is an adaptation of single cells to toxic or life-threatening environments that long preceded organized ani-mal or plant life. Cancer researchers speak of "genomic instability" preceding the pathological cell changes characteristic of cancer.[5] Once mutations have occurred and cancerous cells have started off on their course, it is unlikely that cooperativity could ever be reestablished. The organism must reassert its control over the cells within it, or acquiesce and die.

Preventing and Dealing with Cancer

We have within us millions of genetic triggers that can go off if our cells become chronically unhappy. While this sounds ominous, there are many signals that our cells send out long before they take the drastic step of cancerous growth. With reasonable self-observation, we can detect many of them.

Chronic irritation of our tissues can cause cancer. In rural Kashmir, for example, people hang around their necks a kangri, a clay warming pot with a live coal inside. Skin irritation that results from the heat and rubbing of the kangri over years is ignored, with a skin cancer known as kangri-burn cancer resulting.[6] In eastern Africa, a similar type of cancer of the abdominal wall is associated with the habitual practice of placing warming pans of charcoal directly against the body.[7] In India, habitually chewing betel nuts, a mild but addictive hallucinatory drug that irritates the mucosal lining of the cheek, is associated with cancer of the mouth.[8] These clear associations of behavior predisposing individuals to cancer are the more obvious because of the otherwise very low incidence of cancer in these populations.

When we look at the possible predisposing irritants to which people in the industrialized parts of the world are exposed, the list seems endless (see Table 5). Because there are so many possible car-cinogens, establishing direct causation is frequently difficult. A number of the specific irritants associated with lung, reproductive system, and digestive system cancers will be discussed in following chapters, but tobacco use deserves a particular mention. People who habitually use tobacco ignore the many signs of cellular damage—from smoker's cough to aging skin. Because there are so many potential carcinogenic factors in the industrialized West, it is possible to rationalize the use of tobacco as nonharmful or even benign (as a weight-loss strategy, for example). But tobacco use and any other practices that systematically damage the cellular envi-ronment via chemical, mechanical, or radiation means can and do cause cancer.

Tissues that present large surface areas to potentially damaging carcinogens are predictably at risk. Thus, the digestive system, which comes into contact with virtually every molecule that enters the body from the external environment, is particularly prone to cancer. By some estimates, between 20 percent and 60 percent of all cancers in the United States are related to dietary and nutritional factors.[9] All diets with high contents of fruits, vegetables, and fiber, moderate amounts of fats and carbohydrates, and low amounts of sugar and alcohol are very efficacious in preventing cancer. Single nutrient supplements, such as vitamin C or folate (see chapter 14), are less effective in cancer prevention than adequate amounts of these and other nutrients in an overall good diet.

Avoiding obvious sources of damaging radiation, primarily sunburn for light-skinned people, is an important preventive behavior
for skin cancer, particularly melanoma.

Screening for cancer is a secondary but important preventive
measure. When tumors can be detected and removed early, there
are excellent chances of recovery from cancer. You know your
body better than anyone else, and if you notice changes that may
be indicative of disease you should act on your observations. Your
doctor has age-specific recommendations for screening tests, and
you should schedule a physical examination by your doctor every
two or three years. Keep in mind, however, that doctors are
trained primarily to treat sick people, not people with no symptoms who want to keep from getting sick. Insist on answers and
stick to your guns if you believe that something needs to be
checked out. Change doctors if you must. You are ultimately
responsible for maintaining the evolved homeostasis of your body.

What happens if you get cancer? First, realize that cancers are
common and that survival rates have continued to climb for virtually all cancers detected early. Research your particular type of cancer and find out what the prognosis is. Cancers are classified on the
basis of the type of cells that have begun to proliferate and their
chances of spreading—whether they are quiescent and "benign,"
or aggressive and "malignant."

Treatment for benign cancers is frequently minimal. A tumor
such as an osteoma—an overgrowth of bone—may be removed
surgically for cosmetic reasons, but it will almost certainly not
develop into a life-threatening condition. Malignant tumors, however, may aggressively grow, spreading by both direct cell
encroachment and through natural conduits in the body—the
lymph vessels, the circulatory system, and tissue planes. Its spread
is termed "metastasis."

To stop cancer from spreading and after surgery to remove a
tumor, oncology specialists attempt to kill dividing cells in your
body. You need cell division to stay alive, but not as much as the
cancer does. The idea is to poison or irradiate the cancer cells so
that they are wiped out. In the meantime, you suffer in those areas
where there is a naturally high cell turnover rate—in your gastrointestinal tract (you get nausea) and in your hair (which falls

out because the root cells are killed). Finding a balance between killing the cancer and lessening the physiological impact on you has been the goal of medical oncology, and great strides have been made since the early days of cancer treatment. No other cancers demonstrate these advances more clearly, and how their treatments have interacted with effective prevention and early detection, than breast and reproductive cancers, the subject of the next chapter.

6

Breast Cancer, Prostate Diseases, and Cancers of the Reproductive System

Before humans evolved their complicated nervous system, they developed hormones, which also transport information around the body, but via the blood. These chemicals attach to receptors on target cells and activate them, increasing their metabolic activity, causing them to divide, prompting them to release their secretions, and, if the hormones are produced in so great an abundance that the target cells become too active, causing uncontrolled cell growth, or cancer. In this chapter, we will investigate the latter function in particular: how the communication that's evolved between deposits of fat and breasts, as well as the sex organs, has in the modern Western world caused the two most common cancers—breast cancer among women, and prostate cancer among men.

Hormone Evolution

Hormones are ancient. They date back to the beginning of multicellular organisms (Level 3). The hormone glucagon, for example, which we discuss in chapter 9, evolved between 1 billion and 800,000 years ago, when our ancestors were protoworms.[1] We know this because glucagon is a peptide hormone, composed of amino acids that can be sequenced and counted, and the sequences give us the data to deduce glucagon's evolutionary pathways and time of origin.

Nonpeptide hormones, such as estrogen and testosterone, are steroids, also ancient but not so clearly dated as to their time of origin. However, indicative of their antiquity, estrogen stimulates egg laying in snails and ovary development in shrimp.[2] Amazingly, the hormone has very similar reproductive functions in humans, over a billion years after our divergence from the invertebrates!

A major part of the reason for the remarkable stability of steroid hormones over time is that evolution, rather than altering the hormones themselves, has concentrated on changing the enzymes that act on these basic molecules to produce new hormonal actions.[3] Starting with the precursor of steroid hormones—cholesterol—a P-450 enzyme in the liver (so-named because it is a protein that absorbs light maximally at 450 nanometers) evolved some 800 million years ago to alter it to pregnenolone. Some time later, but before about 700 million years ago, another enzyme evolved that changed pregnenolone to progesterone, still an important human female sex hormone. A cascade of enzymes evolved, in now long-forgotten ancestors before our divergence from invertebrates, that changed precursor steroid molecules to estradiol, the most important estrogen and our other major female sex hormone. In the same time frame, another enzymatic pathway evolved that resulted in the formation of testosterone, the major male sex hormone.

The antiquity of our steroidal hormone system has an important implication for us today. Because these adaptations go back to our very birth as complex organisms, all of our cells are potentially capable of producing sex hormones. Certainly, in the intervening half a billion years, specialized glands such as the ovaries and testes have evolved that concentrate these activities. But recent research utilizing very sensitive radioimmunoassays have shown that fat cells (adipocytes), adrenal gland cells, the liver, and even skin produce significant amounts of estrogens.[4] The enzyme aromatase is responsible for this "peripheral" production of estrogens. These new discoveries about some of our most ancient adaptations provide some key elements in understanding breast cancer.

The Genesis of Breast Cancer

Cancer of the breast in women affects the linings of the ducts that conduct milk from milk-producing lactiferous glands to the nipple. Normally, these cells grow to make the ducts wider and thicker, under the influence of the hormone estrogen, secreted by the ovaries and the placenta during pregnancy. But in cancer, the cells just continue to proliferate, encroaching on other tissue and eventually spreading to other parts of the body.

Who gets breast cancer, and when and where do they get it? Human females born without ovaries do not get breast cancer. Women in traditional societies who have large families do not get breast cancer. Breast cancer occurs most often in women living in Western industrialized societies who are between the ages of 35 and 70. It is most common in overweight women. Breast cancer is the most common form and the deadliest of all cancers affecting women. One in six American women is estimated to be affected. You might think that breast cancer does not affect men, but it does, and although its incidence is much lower, it is just as aggressive a disease.

On first sight, these various epidemiological observations on breast cancer seem puzzling. Females without ovaries do not develop breast cancer because their bodies produce little or no estrogen—the hormone that causes breast tissue to proliferate. But why should hunter-gatherer women, who have had multiple pregnancies and breast-fed their infants, be protected from the disease when Western industrialized women are not?

S. Boyd Eaton, M.D., and colleagues have provided an evolutionary explanation for the high rate of breast cancer in Western women.[5] They suggest that Western women subject their breast tissue cells to much higher levels of estrogen. Because of longer time spent in education, early entry into the job market, older age at marriage, and continuing career pressures, Western women get pregnant for the first time later in life, then have fewer subsequent pregnancies than they used to. Their bodies go through many more menstrual cycles, with their high peaks of estrogen, never balanced by the other primary female sex hormone produced in abundance during pregnancy, progesterone. Non-Western traditional women are, during their reproductive years, usually either producing milk for their suckling infants, when their estrogen levels are also low, or pregnant, when their high estrogen levels are mediated by progesterone. Progesterone, among its other effects, slows down breast cell proliferation. There is an estimated 100-fold difference in North American and hunter-gatherer rates of breast cancer. Social groups in between, such as West Africans (one-twelfth that of North Americans) and the Japanese (one-fourth that of North Americans) have lower rates based on their reproductive patterns. As Japanese women become more like North Americans in having late first pregnancies, they are expected to suffer from a higher rate of breast cancer.

The importance of balancing estrogen and progesterone was discovered independently by the makers of birth control pills, which work by maintaining the body in a high-estrogen state of the early menstrual cycle. Estrogen-only birth control pills contribute to breast cancer, whereas combination estrogen-progesterone birth control pills are not associated with increased risk of breast cancer.

This pattern of delayed first pregnancy and increased spacing between births is exacerbated by the production of estrogens in the body by the "adipose organ"—fat deposits. Western women, as well as men, have been increasing in weight and percentage of body fat, alarmingly so, during the 20th century. In an 18-year period of time, between 1973 and 1991, the World Health Organization (WHO) recorded an increase of 9 percent in the number of obese women in the United States (from 16 percent to 25 percent of women). The current estimate of obese black women in the United States is 49 percent.[6] The relatively greater body fat in girls in Western industrialized societies has effected a full 2-year advancement in the age of menarche—the time when girls have their first menstrual period. This adds 2 years to the high estrogen levels produced by ovarian estrogen after menarche.

To produce estrogen in high amounts, the body must have not only the factories—the ovaries and adipose tissue—but the raw materials. An ancient steroid compound with which we are all selves and simply grow on the peritoneal wall inside the abdominal cavity. But it is a condition in which estrogen stimulates uterine cell growth inappropriately. During the first part of the menstrual cycle, the endometrium normally grows thick under the influence of estrogen, and it is then sloughed off at menstruation as progesterone levels peak. This sloughing off of the endometrial lining of the uterus constitutes the phenomenon of menstrual bleeding. If estrogen levels stay high, endometrial tissue becomes too abundant. Endometriosis may be considered a "precancer" in the sense that its cells are proliferating out of sync with the body but are not yet wildly out of control. Cervical cancer, the sixth most common form of cancer in women, occurs when the endometrial cells begin multiplying, out of control, under the influence of high estrogen levels. Symptoms may be low abdominal pain and bleeding from the vagina.

High levels of estrogen that cause cancer in hormone-sensitive tissues in women also cause cancer in men. Surprisingly, the mechanism is the same, even if the organs and sites affected are different.

Prostate Enlargement and Cancer

The prostate gland is a walnut-size anatomical structure that sits directly below the urinary bladder and in front of the rectum in men. It surrounds the urethra, the tube through which urine passes from the bladder to the outside. Most men are only aware of their prostate gland when it becomes enlarged and begins to block the flow of urine. But the prostate is not a part of the urinary system. Rather, it developed from embryonic gut tissue (endoderm) and developed into a gland of the male reproductive system. Ducts from the prostate enter the urethra and carry the secretory product of the prostate—prostatic fluid. Prostatic fluid is one of the main constituents of semen, the fluid that exits the urethra during male ejaculation.

The exact function of the prostate gland has always been a bit mysterious. Prostatic fluid is not needed for sperm to fertilize eggs in a test tube, but in life this milky fluid may be important during fertilization by providing a medium through which sperm can swim

familiar—cholesterol—is the substrate for sex hormones.
Western diets, as we know, account for a surfeit of this co
in our bodies. We will implicate cholesterol in promo
worsening coronary artery disease (see chapter 7), but it
equally injurious in the genesis of hormonally related canc
as breast cancer.

Another confusing aspect of the data on breast cancer w
women past menopause—the time when the ovaries cease
duce significant levels of estrogen—come down with breast
in significant numbers. Recent research has shown that in
women, estrogen levels are quite high, maintained by prod
of the hormone in adipose tissue around the body.[7] Overw
women, with an excess of adipose tissue, have the highest r
breast cancer after menopause.

Breast cancer in men is also in large part explained by
nonovarian production of estrogen. Overweight men subject
metabolically inactive and residual breast tissue to the prolifera
influence of estrogen, and the malignant cells, although startin
a small mass, aggressively grow and can metastasize throughout
body. Mortality in men from breast cancer, once it becomes est
lished, is proportionately as high as it is in women.

Other Estrogen-Related Reproductive Diseases in Women

High levels of estrogen might be expected to cause other cancers i
target reproductive tissues, such as the ovaries and uterus. Ovaria
cancer, the third most common cancer in women (after breast an
lung cancer), increased in the latter 20th century, as women's fa
deposits increased.[8] But the ovary is somewhat less sensitive to
estrogen than the breast, since it produces the hormone itself and
is not subject to periodic metabolic changes caused by estrogen.

Endometriosis is a condition in which the uterine inner wall,
the endometrium, grows thick and then spreads into the fallopian
tubes. Endometrial cells can even drip through them into the
abdomen, seeding growths of out-of-place uterine tissue that can
become painful during the high-estrogen phase of the menstrual
period. Endometriosis is not cancer because the cells stay to them-

to their eventual destination—an ovary—through the vagina, the uterus, and the fallopian tubes. At puberty the prostate begins to grow under the influence of the hormones testosterone and estrogen, produced by the male gonad, the testis (where sperm are made and released). The prostate remains a hormone-sensitive sex gland throughout life.

Many men in the age range of 50 to 80 years in the industrialized West suffer from an enlargement of the prostate gland known as benign prostatic hyperplasia (BPH). One estimate is that 75 percent of men over age 60 suffer from BPH.[9] They have symptoms of slow urinary flow and sometimes an uncomfortable sense of urgency to urinate.

Many reasons have been advanced for the increase in the number of cells and the increase in size of the prostate gland in BPH. Some medical theorists (mostly men) have suggested that the condition is caused by not enough sex, but no good evidence exists to show that prostatic fluid builds up to cause a medical problem because of few or no ejaculations. Prostatic fluid is simply resorbed by the prostate. Some epidemiological evidence exists that shows a correlation between smoking and prostate cancer, implicating the oxygen free radicals and other carcinogens in cigarette smoke that get into the bloodstream. But the link is not strong, with about the same amount of correlation as other unhealthy behaviors, such as excessive alcohol consumption.

Most theories on the origins of BPH now focus on the finding that prostate cells have receptors for both sex hormones, testosterone and estrogen (estradiol). The testosterone receptors are there because, during embryonic development and again at puberty, the prostate received hormonal instructions from the testis, the male gonad, to enlarge as part of the growth of the male reproductive system. Estrogen receptors are present because estrogen is also an important hormone promoting growth of tissues, even (surprisingly to some) in males. Adolescent human males, for example, have as much estrogen in their bloodstreams as nonpregnant adult women. Theoretically, either an excess of testosterone or an excess of estrogen (or a combination of both) could effect prostate enlargement. Clinical[10] and experimental animal[11] studies indicate that it is an increase in estrogen. But where does the estrogen come from?

Some researchers have implicated the growth hormones fed to beef cattle and other domestic animals that we eat for food as responsible for initiating prostate cancer. Indeed, the European Community has used this reason to ban U.S. beef from its market. No one believes that testosterone (which is metabolized to estradiol in adipose tissue) eaten in beef is good for you, but consistent analyses show that the levels of the hormone, even in two or three steaks a day, are not enough to significantly raise the body's testosterone content above baseline. Until recently, the source of the significant amount of estrogen needed to cause BPH was elusive.

The adipose organ in men—all the aggregate fat tissue in the body—is like the female placenta, an estrogen-producing organ that comes and goes (or at least has the potential to do so). Insights from postmenopausal, obese women who develop breast cancer have helped to solve the mystery. American men have ballooned more than a dozen pounds over the past 50 years, and the weight gain has not been from increased muscle mass or higher stature. Just as in females, male adipose tissue converts cholesterol, the steroid product of fat metabolism in the body, to estradiol. Estradiol in turn binds to receptors on prostate cells and makes them grow and divide. Interestingly, one of the parts of the prostate that estradiol seems to affect most is the caudal lobe (the lowest part of the gland), which contains the prostatic utricle. This normally small part of the prostate, left over from early embryonic development, is homologous to the female vagina and uterus, explaining why it may contain abundant estrogen receptors. Cholesterol levels for obese men have also shot up over the same time period. Thus, exactly the same enlarged adipose organ and abundant supply of precursor that produced estrogen from cholesterol in overweight women, causing breast cancer, exists in obese men, causing prostate enlargement. Prostate cancer, the number one cancer among American men, can be a result of untreated BPH. A large body of clinical evidence indicates that extended exposure of the prostate to elevated estrogen in the blood, in the relative absence of testosterone, is permissive, if not causative, of prostatic cancer. The relative increase in estrogen generated from fat is made even greater as men age and the testes produce less testosterone.

If the most common cancers in both men and women have common causes, is there a common solution to preventing them?

Signs, Symptoms, Treatment, and Prevention

When one arrives at an airport in a country in which the Western industrialized diet—that is, McDonald's, pizza, chips, and Snickers bars—is eaten, the large girth of the majority of the people is striking. Take a trip to Asia, Africa, or the Caribbean, and then return to North America and most of western Europe, and notice the difference. Epidemiologists have noticed the same thing, and they have correlated it with increased levels of cancer. People with lower body weights have much lower incidences of hormone-related cancers. Lowering fat content in your body simply is the best way to avoid reproductive cancers.

In the past, surgery for breast cancer and prostate cancer have loomed as objects of fear for patients suffering from these diseases. Both of these procedures alter the most intimate self-identities of women and men—disfigurement of a part of a woman's body closely connected to her aesthetic and sexual self-image, and impotence in men, an emasculating inability to achieve an erection. If breast cancer and prostate cancer were not so deadly, many would undoubtedly choose to forgo surgery and its aftermath.

Great strides have been made in medical approaches to breast cancer. Radical "mastectomies," in which the entire breast and its underlying muscle are removed, now are rarely done. "Lumpectomies" are much more limited removals of tumor masses from the breast, leaving only a small scar. Carefully monitored chemotherapy and/or radiation therapy control the proliferation of any remaining cancerous tissue in the breast. The earlier a mass can be detected, the less radical the treatment and the greater the chance of survival. Frequent breast self-examination and taking immediate action when a lump is found can result in total recovery from breast cancer.

Men who have had prostate surgery suffer from erectile dysfunction ("impotence") because the prostatic plexus of nerves, located below the gland itself, are cut during surgery. These nerves are autonomic nerves from the sacral vertebrae that cause the erectile tissue of the penis to fill with blood and expand. When they are cut, Viagra (sildenafil citrate) is one solution. This drug replaces the nitric oxide that nerve endings normally supply to the smooth muscle in the erectile bodies of the penis to make them relax and fill with blood during an erection.

Another solution is catching prostate cancer early enough so that only the diseased part of the gland needs to be surgically removed. Most of the gland and the prostatic plexus then remain intact, with few or no problems with erectile dysfunction. A prostate examination, which takes about a minute, should be part of every man's regular physical examination. A laboratory test on a blood sample for prostate specific antigen (PSA), produced when prostate cells have begun to be damaged by cancer, is another preventive measure.

This chapter has laid out an argument for the common causation of hormone-related cancers that is tied to fat—serious diseases related to the increased levels of obesity in people living Western lifestyles. Fat has reached toxic levels in our bodies. But this is not just fat that we eat, it is fat that is stored. Stored fat can be produced from a number of biochemical pathways from foods that we eat. So, if you are overweight but rationalize your obesity on the basis that you eat a "low-fat" diet, beware. It is not what you put in your mouth, but what your cells are in contact with, that determines your internal milieu. Regular physical exercise, control of cholesterol levels, and maintaining normal body weight with good muscle mass for your height are the primary ways to avoid hormone-related cancers, in both men and women. A high-protein, low-carbohydrate diet is the type recommended here to help control your weight and provide your body with the necessary nutrients (chapter 14), but a variety of well-planned low-fat or vegetarian diets can be just as beneficial.

7

Heart Disease and High Blood Pressure: A Story of Fish and Chips

Although it seems counterintuitive, understanding heart disease, the number one killer of people in the industrialized world, depends on understanding the evolution of the kidney. Constant and high-pressure supplies of blood are as important to our kidneys as to our brains. While the brain uses its abundant blood supply to carry on our conscious functions as well as unconscious (autonomic) activities, the kidneys remove waste products, but they also maintain the correct balance of water and circulating chemicals and minerals in our bodies. Our relationship to one class of these chemical compounds—salt—is an adaptation that goes back to our life as fish in the primeval seas. It holds the key to understanding heart disease.

The Evolution of the Kidney and Salt Balance

When our fish ancestors lived in the early seas, the water was much less saline that it is today. The water inside our then-fish bodies was at equilibrium with the surrounding water; that is, dissolved minerals ("salts") were at the same concentrations on the insides and the outsides of our cells. We not only ingested seawater directly but breathed it, extracting oxygen via our gills.[1]

The ancestors of most modern fish and terrestrial vertebrates left the seas for freshwater about 400 million years ago, as we saw in chapter 2. Their physiology then had to evolve to keep the right amount of salt inside their cells, a concentration to which they were, and we still are, adapted. Each of our cells is, in a sense, a droplet of Silurian seawater. Cells also had to keep excess water out, because a higher salt content inside the cell pulls in water to dilute the salt, expanding the size of the cells dangerously. Cells maintain salt-water equilibrium by tiny molecular pumps in their cell membranes that spit out water and gulp in sodium and potassium, the salt molecules. They have a shutoff valve that kicks in when internal salt concentrations are at the right level—that level having been determined by evolution to the environment in which the cell and its surrounding body is adapted.

The situation facing our ancient lobe-finned fish ancestors who moved upstream from the sea can be appreciated by a modern aquarium parable. Let's say that you have an aquarium at home populated by freshwater-adapted goldfish and guppies. A clueless family member who wants to make a surprise addition to the family fish menagerie goes to a pet shop, buys a beautiful coral reef fish, brings it home, and drops it into the aquarium. The poor fish, adapted to seawater, immediately starts to gasp as its overwhelmed cells begin to swell with water and then burst. In a short time the fish floats to the surface—dead. Unlike this unfortunate fish, our early fish ancestors moving into freshwater had cells that could pump out the water rushing in through their cell membranes, and they survived in the new environment. When the body cells of the Silurian lobe-finned fish had adapted to a surrounding low-salt milieu, the excess water expelled from their cells went into the fluid spaces between cells—the so-called extracellular fluid. Now the problem was not the explosion of individual cells from too much water, but too much water in its extracellular "space." Evolution solved this new problem by devising the kidney.

Our original kidney was a segmented affair running on both sides of our spine inside our back, alongside each segmental artery, vein, spinal nerve, and rib. Each kidney unit removed water from our blood and dumped it into the body cavity. From there, little holes called "coelomopores" opened directly to the exterior from which the excess onboard water was jettisoned. The human embryo still has a transient stage (the "pronephros") recalling this ancient adaptation—when we urinated through multiple orifices in our body wall. The system worked very well for millions of years, removing the excess extracellular water extruded by the individual cells of the body. Then animals that had developed a tube connecting the separate kidney units evolved. The so-called mesonephric ("middle") kidney had the advantage of keeping urine out of the body cavity and dumping it via the two long mesonephric ducts out of the hind end of the body. This system is a little more familiar to us. At least there was a single orifice low down on our body through which we urinated. It just happened to be a common one—the cloaca—through which we also defecated and deposited our sex cells.

In one of the most surprising turnarounds in our evolution, the mesonephric ducts, which had conducted urine during the Paleozoic era, evolved to conduct sperm during the Mesozoic. The middle kidney lost its tubular connections to its own ducts and then degenerated over almost its entire length. Its ducts hooked up instead to the male gonads, the testes, and became the vas deferens. Our kidneys, the third and last kidney form to develap, are known as the "metanephros" ("great kidney") and develop as far away from the testes as possible, at the very bottom of the body near the cloaca. These paired organs then ascend deep to our back muscles and outside our gut cavity to a location just below our lowest ribs. They are connected to the blood supply by direct branches off the aorta, the renal arteries. Veins throughout our body pick up the excess extracellular water in our tissues and deliver it to the blood supply, where the heart pumps it around to the kidneys. In the kidneys, blood enters tiny filtering tangles of blood vessels and tubules called the "glomeruli" ("balls of wool"), from which it emerges into an elaborate system of tubules and collecting ducts that selectively take water, salts, and wastes out of the blood. What is left after this process is urine, which then drains down our ureters to our bladder and then out of our body via a now separate opening, the urethra. We are most aware of the kidney's waste disposal function, but maintaining the appropriate balance of water and minerals in the blood is just as crucial.

The evolution of the kidney and its ducts is a bit like the development of plumbing in an old European castle. In its earliest phase, the solutions were diffuse but effective. Pre-Roman internal plumbing was nonexistent and, like the pronephros, the castle lacked any internal piped conduction system for wastes. During the Roman phase, the castle was fitted with a sewer system, coincidentally called a cloaca, that removed wastes in an effective manner, very much like the mesonephros. Then, finally, internal plumbing came, and a water closet, a specialized and dedicated location for waste disposal, replaced the open sewer system. Like the metanephros, the modern toilet conferred significant adaptive advantages and health benefits. But despite all the changes in the details of the plumbing, the kidneys have always functioned to keep the body's internal watery milieu constant. This primitive system and how it works are at the root of the disease that kills more Americans than any other—high blood pressure, also known as hypertension.

The Natural History of Hypertension

Much has been written about high blood pressure, hardening of the arteries, congestive heart failure, myocardial infarction, aortic aneurysm, and angina pectoris—all related components of heart disease. Many medical researchers are involved in studying detailed aspects of each of these disease processes, and each has his or her own theory as to what causes heart disease and how to best prevent or treat the symptoms. The benefit of our approach is that we can go back to the evolutionary origins of heart disease and get down to basics. As Aristotle said, "He who sees things from their beginning has the best view of them."

When we first develop high blood pressure, we reverse our early fish evolutionary trail—from freshwater back to the sea. Many modern bony fish actually did this, evolving salt-excreting glands and severely reducing the number of water-filtering glomeruli in their kidneys. Our ancestors, however, left the streams and the lakes for the land, taking their ancient freshwater fish adaptations with them. Today, eating a diet laden with salt is for our cells tantamount to a sodium chloride bath. Our cells sense the high salt levels around them in the extracellular fluid, delivered there by the blood vessels, which pick the salt up from the gut. The sodium channels in the cells are not open because internal salt levels are adequate. Instead, water begins to leave the cells by osmosis across the cell membranes and into the extracellular fluid. Like a freshwater fish reintroduced into the sea, we begin to swell with water. But on land, where gravity helps fluids collect, we develop extracellular swelling, or edema, in all dependent parts of our anatomy.

The excess water collecting in the spaces between our cells diffuses through the permeable walls of small veins, which in turn return the water to the bloodstream. The total volume of blood flowing through our circulatory system enlarges significantly from this excess water. As blood returns to the heart, it stretches the walls of the first chamber it enters, the right atrium. Nerves from the heart send messages to the brain, which responds with commands via the sympathetic nervous system telling the next chamber of the heart, the right ventricle, to contract more forcefully. The heart now begins to work harder in order to pump a larger volume of blood around the body. Blood pressure increases. Physiologists call this "volume-loading hypertension," and it is the predisposing condition to chronic high blood pressure.[2] The heart produces its own regulating hormone (atrial natriuretic peptide, or ANP) that circulates in the blood and communicates to the kidney that it needs to void salt, thus acting to return the blood volume and blood pressure to normal. But if we continue to overload the system with salt, this compensatory mechanism is overwhelmed.

Why is high blood pressure bad? In our fish and other premammalian ancestors, blood circulated around the body at a slow and sluggish rate. But with the hot-blooded and active mammals, more oxygen was needed in the cells and more rapidly circulating blood became necessary. Their arteries, the blood vessels that must sustain the first violent push of blood when the heart contracts, became thicker and more elastic, while their veins, which return deoxygenated blood to the heart after it has lost a lot of its momentum, remained thin walled, like all the blood vessels of fish. Despite their thickness, human arteries suffer microscopic damage from the increased blood pressure. Small tears occur in their internal walls, especially in areas of turbulence near the branching off of smaller arteries. This damage engenders the same sort of immunological response as a cut on your finger—white blood cells (monocytes) and tissue-based macrophages converge on the site to attack any invading microorganisms, and a scab and then scar tissue begin to form, thickening the area of damage. Scabs do not form inside arteries because of the watery environment, and the deposit is of a different consistency. It complexes with calcium and is termed "plaque." This thickening of arteries in response to high blood pressure is the beginning of "arteriosclerosis"—hardening of the arteries.

Experiments with animals show how increased blood pressure harms the insides of our arteries.[3] Researchers at Stanford University increased blood pressure in rabbits and fed them diets known to be conducive to developing arteriosclerosis. The rabbits developed thickened arterial walls in their aortas. In the belief that the high blood pressure was causing excessive movement of the aorta and damaging its internal lining (the "endothelium"), the researchers surgically placed a sort of immobilizing internal bandage on the aorta in some rabbits. These rabbits were then put on the same hypertensive and atheromagenic dietary regime (one promoting the development of plaques, or "atheromas"), but they did not develop thickened arteries in the immobilized sections of their aortas. Here the endothelial damage was reduced by the artificial restraint, and no thickening of the arterial wall or buildup of plaque occurred.

High blood pressure also harms the two organs through which there is the highest rate of blood flow—the brain and the kidneys—both of which receive between 15 percent and 20 percent of the body's circulation at each pump of the heart. When blood pressure is extremely high, the small arteries in the brain, already weakened by damage to their walls, may burst, causing a stroke. When blood escapes from the blood vessels and bathes brain tissue, the brain tissue dies. The small and delicate glomeruli in the kidney are also subject to damage by high blood pressure. When these membranes are damaged, scarring and fibrosis prevent the kidneys from filtering urine effectively.

The "Essential" Nature of Hypertension

It is standard medical opinion that "essential" hypertension, the kind that affects some 95 percent of Americans, is of unknown cause.[4] This idea is mistaken and is a legacy of old physiological research on hypertension. We can deduce the cause of essential hypertension from the overwhelming amount of epidemiological data from around the world that shows that people who eat low-salt diets simply do not have hypertension. Not when they are young. Not when they are old. They do not die of heart disease, except when infections, particularly rheumatic fever caused by streptococcal bacteria, or parasites, as in the African and South American malady of endomyocardial fibrosis, cause in situ heart dysfunction. Only in rare circumstances do people outside the industrialized West die of heart failure. For example, during the month of July in rural northern Nigeria, cardiac failure in women giving birth is relatively high (1 percent of the women in labor).[5] But this unfortunate phenomenon is explicable by environmental conditions and cultural practices: July is the hottest month, the women lie on a bed over a fire during labor, and they are fed salt-rich lake food. From what we have already seen, increasing the cellular salt content leads to an increase in extracellular fluid, which in turn leads to an increase in blood volume and high blood pressure. This extra load on the heart, coupled with loss of water through urination and sweating and the accompanying imbalance in essential electrolytes, especially potassium, can cause heart failure. Overall, however, hypertension "appears to be totally absent from societies described as 'stone age.'"[6]

Generally the diets of these societies are low in saturated fats, low in carbohydrates, high in fiber, and high in many minerals and vitamins, all of which have been thought at one time or another to be equally important in controlling hypertension. So what epidemiological evidence is there to suggest that it is the low salt content of their diet that maintains normal blood pressure? Research by the Swedish biomedical researcher Staffan Lindeberg at Lund University in the Trobriand Islands of the South Pacific is very instructive.[7] Lindeberg measured the blood pressures of rural Kitava people of all ages and found that the population had a negligible amount of hypertension. But in measuring their cholesterol, he found that their readings were nearly off the chart. Islanders eat a lipid-rich diet based on coconuts, but they are physically active and are not obese. Salt in their diet is low. Lindeberg's results make sense only in light of the high-salt hypothesis for the genesis of hypertension. High cholesterol in the bloodstream exacerbates the condition by latterly contributing to plaque formation in arteries but in itself is not a cause of initial hypertension.

Land Vertebrate Aspects of Hypertension

Hypertension is not just a story of fish evolution. Changes that evolved in the vertebrate kidney when our ancestors became land-dwellers made possible the important conservation of water and the further retention of salt—the two essentials that were limited in a subaerial terrestrial environment. The adaptations that evolved in the land-living vertebrates overprinted but did not change the basic nature of the salt-water balance inherited from fish ancestors.

A remarkable multi-organ cooperation took shape in the first land vertebrates, probably labyrinthodont amphibians (our Level 8 ancestors; see chapter 2), in order to conserve salt and water. The kidney produces an enzyme called "renin" when the salt content in the blood and extracellular water volume begin falling. An enzyme speeds up a chemical reaction, and renin acts to enhance the chemical change of a liver hormone, angiotensinogen, to a more rapidly working hormone, angiotensin I. The lungs, which evolved from the swim bladders of our air-breathing fish ancestors, produce another enzyme, angiotensin converting enzyme (ACE), which then acts on angiotensin I to produce angiotensin II. This hormone causes contraction of smooth muscle around small arteries, including those in the kidneys, decreasing the rate at which blood flows through and is filtered by the kidney. Thus, by this remarkable interactive process, which involves kidneys, liver, lungs, and heart, water is filtered out of the blood and salt is conserved.

Another organ, the suprarenal (or adrenal) gland sitting atop the kidney, also comes into the act. Renin in the blood also stimulates the suprarenal gland to produce aldosterone, a steroid hormone that makes the kidney reabsorb salt from its urine. These adaptations are all related to conserving water and salt in a terrestrial environment. Although the terrestrial adaptations of the kidney are not the key to the origins of hypertension, they did provide the first scientific advances into understanding its exacerbation. In the 1920s, the physiologist Harry Goldblatt surgically reduced the blood flow of the renal arteries in a dog, thus artificially reducing the blood flow to its kidneys. The kidneys reacted as if water were suddenly in short supply (and blood volume consequently reduced), because this was the body's evolved reaction. "Vasoconstriction," the tightening of smooth muscle around arterioles, occurred. Goldblatt was able to isolate for the first time a "vasoactive substance" in the blood—a hormone we now call "angiotensin." The renin-angiotensin system has been of major clinical importance in the treatment of hypertension because physicians can manipulate it with drugs and the patient's own physiology in bringing high blood pressure down to near-normal limits. How did such a system evolve in the first place?

Surprisingly, the liver produces angiotensinogen, whose original function was probably digestive. We may hypothesize that in the early freshwater fish, as extracellular fluid volume and salt (mainly from ingested food) began to fall, the liver released this substance into the bloodstream, which then caused the kidney to retain both salt and water. Angiotensinogen also acts to close down the diameter of blood vessels in order to conserve resources and reduce blood flow to the body's tissues. We can imagine that the liver produced angiotensinogen when food was scarce and our sluggish fish ancestors became even more sluggish in order to wait out a drought or similar lull in resources. African lungfish, for example, can live quiescent for months in a dried-out clump of mud, reducing their heart rate to about three beats per minute.[8]

Our kidneys are not exactly the same as early freshwater fish kidneys. A significant change happened about 340 million years ago when our ancestors, the lobe-finned fish, began crawling out of the water. They may have begun wriggling onto dry land on their fleshy fins in order to escape predators, or to escape drying pools and find other bodies of water in which they could survive. They and their descendants, the amphibians and reptiles, became increasingly independent of water, neither requiring it to complete their reproductive cycle nor to find food. When life on land evolved, there was no longer a surfeit of water surrounding the body, although the cells maintained their ancient seawater environment. The kidneys now needed to adapt to reabsorbing water so it would not be lost to excretion. The elongated loops of the kidney tubules evolved to be able to take in water and concentrate the urine.

Another major physiological change happened when animals moved out of the water and onto land—they started breathing air. The lungs also come into the hypertension act by producing angiotensin converting enzyme, which speeds up the transformation of angiotensin I to angiotensin II, a very powerful contractor of the smooth muscle around arterioles. ACE is found in living air-breathing fish,[9] but it was the evolution of the lung that saw the major elaboration of this enzyme. ACE allowed the lungs of the first amphibians and reptiles living on land to respond to a drop in blood pressure in the lungs by stimulating constriction of the body's blood vessels, thereby causing a rise in overall blood pressure.

Hypertension from Stress

Stress—pain, fear, and trauma—also affects blood pressure. Blood pressure rises in stressful situations and more blood is supplied to the skeletal muscles to run away or fight. The brain assesses stress and now comes into physiological interaction with the other organs affecting hypertension. The brain uses two methods to communicate—hormones released in the blood and received by distant organs, and nerves, hard-wired between the central nervous system and the peripheral parts of the body. The pituitary, a gland at the base of our brain, produces a hormone called "vasopressin," formerly called "antidiuretic hormone," which in turn causes the kidney to reabsorb water and thus raise blood pressure. Autonomic nerve fibers connecting to the hypothalamus, which is sometimes called the "head ganglion" of the sympathetic nervous system, also affect our blood pressure and heart rate. The sympathetic system, referred to as the "fight-or-flight" nervous system, increases heart rate, opens up blood supply to skeletal muscle, and decreases blood supply to the gut. Sympathetic nerves also cause epinephrine (also called "adrenaline") to be released from the suprarenal ("adrenal") gland into the bloodstream. Epinephrine increases heart rate and blood pressure.

Stress is hard to measure, and its effects in raising blood pressure may be more episodic than the constant effect of raised salt levels in the diet. Studies do show that stress and other psychological forces, such as hopelessness (as demonstrated in a recent study of Finnish men), act to increase the likelihood of heart disease. This worsening effect is added to the underlying essential hypertension already present in many societies.

A newly discovered hormone called "adrenomedullin" is produced by the suprarenal gland from a precursor hormone that comes from the pituitary gland. This hormone acts to relax the smooth muscle around arterioles and thus counteracts the effects of sympathetic innervation as well as vasopressin, both of which are vasoconstrictors and increase blood pressure.

The Results of Hypertension

Some researchers believe that hardening of the arteries—the deposits of cholesterol and free fatty acids of plaque on the insides of the arteries—is the primary and underlying cause of hypertension. The constriction of the diameter of the arteries, they think, causes faster blood flow and makes the heart pump harder. But evidence shows raised blood pressure alone accounts for the thickening of arteries.[10] Plaque deposits only build up on roughened and damaged sections of arteries. The fatty streaks that even the arteries of American children and teenagers are beginning to show are formed over endothelium that has been damaged by high blood pressure. It is true that relatively few teenagers are found to be hypertensive when tested with a standard blood pressure cuff, but at this early stage of hypertension there is a reflexive, constrictive response of the small blood vessels that hides the high incipient hypertension. Small blood vessels throughout the body, particularly the arterioles, contract in response to the higher blood pressure. A doctor cannot detect a rise in blood pressure, but that negative finding may be illusory. An apparently "normotensive" person may in fact be like a car in gear with the brakes on—moving forward, but slowly, and with a significant amount of mechanical strain.

There has been a tremendous amount of public attention paid to cholesterol and its role in causing arteriosclerosis. People may joke about "coating their arteries" when they eat bacon, ice cream sundaes, and chocolate mousse, but if the image evoked is slathering oil or grease on the inside of a tube, then the metaphor is inappropriate. Our arteries must in fact have a break in their endothelial lining to begin the process of arteriosclerosis. Once this occurs, the process of hardening the arteries is much more akin to a slow growth of bacteria or corrosion, which also begin at small surface defects and then grow.

Heart attack is technically known as an "infarction," a condition resulting from the blockage of blood flow to the muscle of the heart, the myocardium. Interestingly, the heart is just an overgrown contractile artery that twists back on itself during embryological development. The blood that it pumps does not supply any oxygen to its muscular walls. Small arteries that branch off from the aorta—the coronary arteries, so named because they form a crown around the heart—curve around the heart to supply its muscle. Because of the extremely high pressures that build up in the aorta in hypertension, the coronary arteries become damaged. They clog up with arteriosclerotic plaque. Blood flow to the heart is decreased, the myocardial cells begin screaming for oxygen, and pain ("angina pectoris") can result. Bypass surgery can open up the coronary arteries and resupply the myocardium with oxygen, alleviating angina.

Congestive heart failure occurs when the volume of blood entering the heart is too much for the heart muscle to pump out. Blood backs up, either in the lungs or in the peripheral tissues. Fluid builds up in the extracellular space and swollen ankles and hands result. Even more fluid attempts to return to the blood plasma, and blood volume expands even more. Eventually, the overtaxed heart fails.

Bipedalism, Hypertension, and the Brain

Because we hominids adapted to an upright, bipedal posture, the heart has to push blood up into the head with increased force in order to overcome the effects of gravity. The giraffe's heart, because of this species' long neck, has made the same adaptation. This adaptation makes our carotid arteries, the vascular connections from our hearts to our heads, particularly susceptible to damage from high blood pressure. The carotid arteries are a frequent location of arteriosclerosis, and in advanced cases they need to be surgically opened up to allow blood to flow to the brain.

Quadrupedal animals have their heads at the same level as their hearts, along a line more or less parallel to the ground. Humans, on the other hand, have a brain that sits atop a column of blood that has to be pushed up by the heart directly against the pull of gravity into, around, and through the entire head and neck region. Hypertension has the effect of increasing an already increased rate of blood flow to the brain. Consequently, our brain becomes particularly susceptible to stroke, which is a "cerebrovascular accident" such as a clot or a small bleeding defect within the brain.

In evolutionary terms, the human brain has come to occupy an elevated position, both literally and figuratively, and at the same time it is vulnerable to losing its lifeline of blood and oxygen. To be able to communicate its plight should the heart fall down on its job of keeping up a good head of blood pressure, the brain evolved the ability to produce vasopressin, mentioned before in regard to the stress response, to increase blood pressure. This hormone was once called antidiuretic hormone for its mechanism of action—it prevents water loss by urination ("diuresis"), keeps extracellular fluid volume high, and thus maintains high blood volume and blood pressure through affecting the kidney's tubules. The pituitary releases vasopressin into the bloodstream in response to an increase in salt content in the blood as sensed by receptors in the hypothalamus. The secreting cells are near the "thirst center" in the hypothalamus, which drives our desire to drink. A fall in blood pressure as sensed by the nerve receptors in the left atrium of the heart also causes secretion of vasopressin.

An upright, bipedal stance may also help to explain why the descending aorta is virtually always the first site to show evidence of atherosclerotic plaque. The high blood pressure from the heart, pushing blood into the first (the ascending) part of the aorta, has to work against gravity; but once blood turns the corner and heads down the descending aorta, gravity helps to speed its course.

Quadrupedal mammals do not have such a vertical course of the major artery in the body, and the human course of the descending aorta predisposes this part of the aorta to damage from high blood pressure.

When the aorta walls thicken from small-scale damage and immunological reaction, they also become weaker. Parts of the endothelium can begin to split off in layers, and high-velocity blood flow can actually begin to peel off sections of aortic wall. The sides of the aorta may begin to bulge dangerously under the pressure. This condition, known as "aortic aneurysm," can become life-threatening if the bulge ruptures.

Why Are African Americans Particularly Susceptible to Hypertension?

Epidemiological surveys consistently demonstrate that African Americans have the greatest per capita incidence of hypertension and heart disease. While the same dietary and exercise factors that cause hypertensive diseases in other populations are undoubtedly at the root of the problem, there does seem to be a disproportionate effect in this population. Thomas Wilson suggested that the largely arid continent of Africa produced in Africans an adaptation of greater kidney resorption of salt than in other populations.[11] He related the high rate of "dropsy" (fluid accumulation) in historic West Indian slave populations to hypertensive heart disease. A diet of salted fish and meat and a high rate of salt use as a condiment were primary causes of hypertension. Another hypothesis attributes the superior salt-retaining abilities of African Americans, which by some measures are higher than in Africans, to the high mortality from salt depletion suffered by this population during transport in slave ships. These genes were passed on to present-day African Americans, perhaps explaining their disproportionate suffering from hypertension.

Whatever the exact evolutionary cause, African Americans do seem to have an adaptation for retaining water and salt, more so than other populations. This physiological attribute helps to explain a tendency toward hypertension in this population, as well as differences in the actions of antihypertensive drugs. Although the precise mechanisms are still unclear, two otherwise popular prescription medications for hypertension—ACE inhibitors, such as captopril and enalapril; and beta-blockers, such as acebutolol and propanolol—are not as effective in African Americans compared to most other patients.

Preventing and Treating Hypertension from an Evolutionary Perspective

Low-salt diets among hunter-gatherers are responsible for the lack of high blood pressure in these groups. The incidence of hypertension also does not increase with age in hunter-gatherers, unlike people in the modern West. Extrapolation from the diets of modern hunter-gatherers and from the paleoanthropological record indicates that our evolved normal intake of sodium is 1 gram per day. Instead, we eat between 9 to 12 grams of salt per day on average. Salt is high in many of the processed and canned foods that we eat. A small bag of potato chips, for example, contains one-third of an entire day's sodium allotment. Consumption needs to be less than a maximum of 4 grams of salt a day to avoid measurable hypertension.[12]

A large-scale clinical study on the dietary aspects of treating hypertension was completed in 1998. The multicenter project was termed "DASH" ("Dietary Approaches to Stop Hypertension"). The DASH program includes seven to eight servings of grains, eight to ten servings of fruits and vegetables, and three servings of low-fat dairy products daily, and no more than two servings of meat and four to five servings of legumes and nuts per week. Salt in the DASH diet is between 1.5 and 3.0 grams per day. The DASH diet differs from the Paleolithic diet (see chapter 14), but it shares many of the same attributes. The DASH diet has proved as effective as drugs in the control of hypertension. Dietary modification coupled with exercise is by far the best therapy for hypertension.

Pharmacological remedies—"medicines"—act to intervene in one or another physiological process and thereby restore our body's equilibrium when we are sick. As we have seen in earlier chapters, our evolutionary perspective gives us a guide to help decide which pharmaceutical approach may be the least damaging to the body's intrinsic operating principles, and thus more acceptable to us. In the realm of heart medications—the largest single group of drugs, except for pain relievers, used by Americans—some guidance is important.

There are four broad categories of antihypertensive drugs: (1) diuretics, which promote urination and reduction of extracellular fluid, thus reducing the "preload" of the heart and reducing blood pressure; (2) beta-blockers, which confuse the receptors on heart muscle cells for sympathetic nerve stimulation, thus reducing heart contractions; (3) ACE inhibitors, which block the effect of angiotensin converting enzyme from the lungs in the last step of activating angiotensin, thus reducing smooth muscle contractions of arterioles and the "peripheral resistance" of the circulatory system, a major mechanical determinant of blood pressure; and (4) calcium channel blockers, which reduce the amount of the element calcium in the heart muscle cells, thus reducing their ability to contract.

Considering that the primary problem in hypertension is too much water in the extracellular space, the first remedy that physicians prescribe for hypertension is a drug that causes urination—a diuretic. Diuretics act at the level of kidney tubules, preventing the reabsorption of sodium, thus blocking part of the adaptation that land-living animals made to retain water and sodium. From an evolutionary perspective, reducing the amount of extracellular fluid and blood volume is the most basic solution to the problem of hypertension. Because diuretics act at this most recent level of evolution and also are sited at primarily one location in the body, the kidney tubules, they are generally effective. But they also have significant side effects, such as a general loss of potassium and other electrolytes, along with sodium, from the body.

Beta-blockers directly decrease heart rate by interacting with beta-receptor molecules in heart muscle and by reducing the release of renin by the kidney. They thus interrupt not only the salt-water balance mechanisms underlying hypertension, but the stress response mediated by the sympathetic nervous system. Beta-blockers do not solve the problem of excess extracellular fluid and must be used with diuretics.

ACE inhibitors turn back the evolutionary clock to the hour of the pre-lobe-fin fish (Level 7A), blocking the action of the last-evolved enzyme in the angiotensin pathway, angiotensin converting enzyme, produced in the lung. These drugs do not work well in African Americans, a Level 17 phenomenon.

Calcium channel blockers hamper the participation of calcium in the contraction of smooth muscle and cardiac muscle. In comparison with the other antihypertensive drugs, they derange a more basic and systemwide physiological function, the contraction of all the body's smooth muscle. They do reduce blood pressure, but, not surprisingly, they have significant negative side effects on other body systems, such as the digestive system. These drugs are also associated with a higher rate of heart failure because they actually decrease the ability of the heart muscle to contract.

It is worth emphasizing that a DASH-style or low-salt diet and a moderately active lifestyle—characteristics of our evolutionary past—are behavioral modifications with no side effects that prevent hypertension and its sequelae. Eating within our adaptively central zone will protect us generally against high blood pressure and heart disease. Such a simple solution seems too easy and too low-tech for such a widespread scourge. Fully effective medicines or genes wholly responsible for hypertension will not be found because the condition is a result of discordance between our evolutionary past and our present lifestyles. A cure for our epidemic of heart disease lies in the realm of large-scale behavioral modification, perhaps one of humankind's greatest challenges simply because it is so basic and so immune to technological solutions.

8

Why We Smoke

Smoking causes cancer. Only recently would most people agree with this statement. Convincing epidemiological data from Germany in the 1920s, as well as many later studies, linking smoking and lung cancer were widely ignored. Strong economic interests opposed the identification and recognition of the disease-causing properties of tobacco. After all, the tobacco industry was what gave the American colonies their first global economic clout, and well-ensconced commercial interests mounted massive marketing campaigns for smoking. But economics and marketing alone do not explain the widespread popularity of smoking and use of tobacco. We must look to evolutionary origins to understand why people are drawn to and then persist in using a substance that so consistently kills them.

Hydrocarbons and Lung Cancer

Lab rodents and nonhuman primates can be trained to self-administer nicotine, but smoke itself is rarely a substance to which they become accustomed or which they will self-administer. Humans, on the other hand, like smoke. We preserve foods, such as ham, fish, and other meats, by smoking them. We barbecue over an open fire for the flavor of the smoke. We even artificially flavor food with smokiness, such as barbecue-flavored potato chips. We light our fireplaces, campfires, and incense just to smell the smoke. And finally, some of us inhale a variety of aromatic tobaccos in pipes, cigars, and cigarettes.

With the exception of smoking, exposing ourselves to a moderate amount of smoke does not seem to have negative health consequences. We have a set of liver enzymes, the cytochrome P-450 monooxygenase enzyme system, that acts to detoxify the hydrocarbons in smoke. All indications are that smoke, in moderate amounts, is a substance to which humans are adapted. As we saw in chapter 2, the use of fire by hominids dates back as far as 1.7 million years ago. We can thus surmise that our P-450 enzymes have evolved over the course of the fire-using part of our evolutionary history.

Why would an attraction to smoke ever evolve? Where there is smoke there is fire, and perhaps a more trenchant question to ask is, what adaptive advantage did the use of fire confer on our ancestors? Whatever selective advantages fire use offered, they had to outweigh the basic eye-irritating and cough-generating physiological side effects. Natural selection performed quite a feat in rendering smoke palatable to us human beings.

Fire is a powerful natural phenomenon that evokes fear and avoidance in virtually all species. For hominids, controlling it gave them immense power over interspecific competitors and prey species alike. Hominids could set a fire on a stretch of savanna, clear out all the large carnivores, and drive the game before the flames. In a one-on-one encounter, a fire-wielding hominid became a formidable foe for any animal. As hominids spread into higher latitudes and ice age climates became colder, fire became ever more important for warmth within shelters and for light. Cooking became a way to render parasite-laden meat safe to eat, toxic plants edible, and tough foods chewable and digestible. The extreme expansion of hominids' niche that fire made possible easily explains why smoke became a "nice" smell. We can surmise that hominids who did not like the smell of smoke statistically found themselves without fire in a critical encounter with a lion, undone by a parasitic infestation, or underfed and weakened when famine struck, and thus unlikely to survive. The evolutionary equation became: where there is smoke there is fire; where there is fire there is safety; where there is smoke there is safety.

To a point. With too much smoke, our eyes water and our lungs scream for fresh air. What explains the addiction of many modern hominids to smoking—something so strong that it overrides our natural physiological defenses—is an evolutionary heritage much more ancient. It began when we and the insects were one, embodied in the same species and sharing the same genes, 1.0 to 1.2 billion years ago (see Table 1).

The Evolutionary Biology of the Tobacco Plant

The wild tobacco plant grows in the ecological riot of the rain forest, where competition among plant species for light, soil, nutrients, and space is intense. Natural selection favors any advantages of growth and reproduction that a species may have. In the case of the relatively slow-growing tobacco plant, a toxic substance in its leaves—nicotine—evolved to deter animals from eating it by making them sick to their stomachs. Chemically, nicotine is an alkaloid, a class of poisons widely distributed in the plant kingdom and evolved in various forms through the ongoing chemical warfare between plants and animals. The main animals to which the tobacco plant evolved this defense were insects, whose small bodies were maximally affected by the toxic effects of the chemical. Nicotine is still used in commercial insecticides. For large animals like humans, the toxic effects of nicotine, unless large amounts are ingested, are much more muted.

Nicotine is a neurotoxin, a chemical that affects nerves. It is picked up by receptors on the surfaces of nerve cells and certain other modified nerve cells throughout the body known as "chemoreceptors." Nicotine substitutes itself for the chemicals that normally attach to the nicotinic receptors, and therefore alters the functions of muscles and nerves. Nicotine causes death by paralyzing the respiratory muscles, thus asphyxiating the insect. If a human being accidentally ingests the same relative amount of nicotine as an insect who munches on a tobacco leaf, he would immediately grow short of breath and his pulse would slow. His skeletal muscles would twitch before becoming paralyzed, and he would die within 10 to 30 minutes.[1]

The "purpose" for which nicotine evolved in the tobacco plant—to kill or at least dissuade insects from eating the plant's leaves—gives it, paradoxically, physiological effects humans perceive as pleasurable. Nicotine constricts blood vessels, increasing the heart rate and thus acting as a stimulant in the body. Because of its muted emetic properties, nicotine also suppresses a smoker's appetite, which makes it, in a twisted way, a diet enhancer. The most important side effect, however, is nicotine's effect on the brain.

Nicotine is a chemical mimic of acetylcholine, one of the major neurotransmitters in the human body. Both release chemicals in the brain, particularly dopamine, from the sensory cortex, the midbrain, and the hippocampus. These parts of the brain are involved in its "reward system" and are implicated in the addiction to many drugs.[2]

The Ethnohistory of Smoking

South American Indians first discovered the pharmacological properties of the tobacco plant, *Nicotiana tabacum*, endemic to the Amazonian rain forest. The plant was dried, rolled into cigars, or ground up to smoke in pipes, usually in ceremonies. Tobacco in high concentrations has a mild hallucinatory effect. But tobacco was also used as an emetic, to induce vomiting, by being eaten directly. American Indians, along with most peoples of the world, have believed in the efficacy of "purgatives" in ridding the body of disease. It is this property of the tobacco plant—its emetic effect—that explains part of the evolutionary origins of the psychoactive substance in tobacco, nicotine.

The psychoactive effects of nicotine conferred an unintended benefit on the plant's geographical dispersal. In pre-Columbian times, Central and North American Indians cultivated the plant for its medicinal and ceremonial properties. *Nicotiana* spread northward from the Amazonian rain forests. It was along the eastern North American seaboard that early Anglo-Americans first encountered tobacco and began growing it for export. Virginia became well known for its tobacco, and profits from its plantations became the manifestation of the New World gold that had originally drawn many European fortune seekers.

The scanty evidence that exists indicates that lung cancer was a rare or nonexistent disease during the thousands of years that American Indians used tobacco, as well as during the three centuries that it was initially smoked in the Old World. Tobacco was largely smoked in pipes, both by Indians and Euro-Americans. In colonial times, clay pipes with long stems were smoked in taverns. The ends of the pipe stems were broken off after each use. And the amount of actual tobacco smoke inhaled was small. For many years, tobacco smoke was even considered by many to be therapeutic, "clearing out" the respiratory passages.

Cigarettes became the favorite mode of tobacco use during and after World War II. These finely shredded leaves of cured tobacco wrapped in paper are innovations from Turkey, which had become a secondary export center for tobacco in the 19th century. The increased surface area of the tobacco and the increased heat with which it burned delivered a hit of nicotine to the vast surface area of the lungs physiologically very different from the slow-burning twists of colonial tobacco. The pick-me-up kick from a cigarette became popular among the GIs at the front, and enterprising tobacco companies supplied millions of free cigarettes as part of the war effort. The volume of carcinogenic smoke inhaled in a single cigarette was vastly more than from a pipe, and multiple cigarettes— a pack of twenty—tended to be chain-smoked. Returning soldiers brought the habit of cigarette smoking back with them from the war. By the 1950s, there was an epidemic of lung cancer in the United States.

Aware of the history of tobacco, it may seem strange that Native American rhetoric blames the white man for the curse of smoking and associated lung disease. But it was in fact the innovation of the Turkish cigarette that transformed smoking from a low-grade irritant into a primary carcinogen.

Lung Cells React: Lung Cancer and Emphysema

Abundant epidemiological research confirms that nicotine is the psychoactive substance in cigarette smoke and the primary reason that smokers light up time and again. Nicotine promotes so much smoking that the amount of carbon-containing tar deposited overwhelms the body's detoxifying systems. Lung cells begin to feel poisoned and betrayed by the body, and they eventually rebel. But nicotine is only one of the substances that causes lung cancer. Cigarette smoke, in addition to nicotine, has many caustic chemical components. By one estimate, the deadly fog inhaled from a lit cigarette is composed of some 150 ingredients, including carbon monoxide, cyanide, and tar. Many can cause cellular injury and thus lead to cancer, but it is probable that tar, a "polycyclic aromatic hydrocarbon" (PAH) formed by unburned but charred tobacco leaf fragments, is the primary culprit.

At the cellular level, pathologists have determined the steps in the development of various forms of lung cancer. Polycyclic aromatic hydrocarbons from partially combusted organic materials—in the case of smokers, tobacco leaf fragments—bathe lung cells. PAHs are metabolized to carcinogens in the body, particularly benzoapyrene, chrysene, and benzoantracene, which react with the DNA in the cell nucleus of lung cells.[3] A number of oncogenes, particularly the *ras* and *myc* genes, become turned on. Mutations occur in the tumor suppressor genes *p53* and *rb*.[4] These genes are the start buttons for cells to begin replicating on their own. They forget that they were once lung cells and regress to their ancient single-minded single-cellness.

The acrid nature of cigarette smoke damages another part of the lungs—the air-exchanging alveoli—and brings on another set of diseases in addition to lung cancer. Broadly described as chronic obstructive pulmonary disease (COPD), they are the fifth-most-common cause of death in the United States. Emphysema lies at the heart of COPD.

Emphysema in human beings is a failure of the heart-lung adaptation of the first air-breathing animals. When lungs evolved in ancient land-living animals, some 340 million years ago, additional chambers of the heart appeared in order to pump blood to the lungs, and at higher pressure. Smoking works against this adaptation by decreasing the ability of the lungs to exchange oxygen and carbon dioxide. In order to compensate, the newly evolved part of the heart—the "right heart"—becomes overworked, enlarged, and thicker walled. Many of the symptoms that we experience in emphysema—sluggishness, breathlessness during exertion, and slowing down of metabolism—represent a regression to preamphibian characteristics.

The many caustic ingredients in cigarette smoke, other than tar, are responsible for emphysema. Experimental animals can be given emphysema by administering to their lungs protein-digesting enzymes such as plant-derived papain (from papayas) or elastase produced by animal pancreas or white blood cells.[5] These substances attack the walls of the small air sacs, the alveoli, in the lungs, enlarging them by eating away the elastin proteins in their cells. Elastase is probably produced by macrophages, agents of the immune system, reacting to carbon or other irritants in cigarette smoke deposited in the lungs. Oxygen free radicals contained in cigarette smoke are another likely cause of cellular damage to the elastic tissue of the alveoli. The alveoli become enlarged, lose their natural rebound, and fail to empty out their air at the end of a breathing cycle. Oxygen levels in the blood begin to fall and carbon dioxide levels begin to rise. Emphysema patients feel out of breath and are unable to exert themselves in even simple tasks.

The heart becomes profoundly affected in COPD. The chemoreceptors in the arterial system sense that carbon dioxide is too high and send neural messages to the brain that are transmitted by the cardiac nerves to increase the heart rate. The heart pumps faster, but the inelastic lungs are not able to deliver any more oxygen to the blood. Eventually, the heart fails from excessive muscle fatigue and a never-ending demand to pump harder. The most common cause of death in COPD and emphysema is congestive heart failure.

Amphibians have a major advantage over the emphysema patient, however. Despite their sluggish blood flow and low rate of gas exchange in the lungs, their moist, thin skin breathes. Our skin has a relatively thick and impervious epidermis, which prevents the wet interior of our body from drying out. Even if we were to crawl under wet leaf litter on the forest floor or hang out under the verdant fronds near mountain streams, it is doubtful if these typical amphibian habitats would help to alleviate our emphysema.

Emphysema is treated by delivering oxygen to the lungs, the idea being that a higher concentration of oxygen in the relatively smaller fraction of air that circulates through the lungs will be enough to sustain the patient. The small portable oxygen tanks and clear plastic tubes snaking bilaterally into a patients' nose as they wheel themselves through shopping malls has become an all-too-familiar sight.

The changes to the alveoli in emphysema are unfortunately irreversible, so the only course to avoid the disease is to prevent it: don't smoke.

Preventing Lung Cancer and Emphysema

Are we captive to our evolved cravings and addictive tendencies, inevitably destined for disease, or is there a way that we can avoid lung cancer, emphysema, and their related deleterious effects?

It is very difficult to stop smoking. You are up against millions of years of evolution once you are addicted to nicotine, and our evolved predilection for smoke reinforces the behavior. Smokers variously describe their addiction as "an old friend," a behavior that relaxes them, a reward, something to do with their hands, oral satisfaction, a part of their personality, or a social statement. To stop smoking usually requires several steps, but a strong desire to change your behavior is paramount and the most important.

The best way to avoid lung cancer and emphysema is not to start smoking. You can engage your evolved predilection for smoke by weekend barbecues, fireplaces, camping out, working in an incense shop, or even signing up as a volunteer fireman. The key to prevention is to embrace the concept of limited exposure to the hydrocarbons in smoke. It is simply outside the evolved capabilities of our bodies to detoxify massive amounts of carbon in our lungs.

But what if you have already become enmeshed in one of the social or physiological traps of smoking. What is the best way to escape?

Smoking is like any other addiction. It demands total loyalty and pushes aside family, friends, and all other responsibilities.

Smoking cessation experts agree that addiction to tobacco must be dealt with just the same as drug or alcohol addictions (chapter 13). A program to stop smoking must include a reorientation of behavior and lifestyle.

Aids in smoking cessation recommended by preventive medicine specialists may help. Nicotine polacrilex gum, which is chewed, and nicotine transdermal patches, which are worn on the skin, were developed based on the realization that nicotine causes the addiction to cigarettes. By dosing yourself with relatively small amounts of nicotine through a different route of administration—the mouth lining or the skin—you can avoid the effects of acrid, hydrocarbon-containing smoke in your lungs. Eventually, by gradually reducing the amount of nicotine administered through the skin patch, you become physiologically less dependent on the drug. But smoking is a complicated behavior, invested with many positive associations, and it is impossible to stop without a great degree of internal personal commitment.[6]

You will tend to gain weight when you stop smoking. This possibility works as a major disincentive for many people to stop smoking. Don't let it happen. At the same time you drop cigarettes, start on a paleodiet and an exercise regime (chapter 14). Eating foods you have evolved to like and getting hooked on endogenous endorphins generated by physical exercise is a lot better than being addicted to nicotine. And this solution not only keeps your weight down, it also significantly lowers blood pressure, increases muscle tone, causes you to sleep better, and reduces stress, not to mention removing the carcinogens in cigarette smoke from your body.

"Chemoprevention" is an approach to avoiding the ill effects of smoking by attempting to counteract specific noxious chemicals in cigarette smoke. A recent suggestion, for example, was made that aspirin and similar NSAIDs (nonsteroidal anti-inflammatory drugs) could effectively block the carcinogenic action of a component of cigarette smoke, NNK, a nitrosamine.[7] Administering vitamin A derivatives, such as retinoic acid or beta-carotene (a vitamin A provitamin), can also help.[8] These forms of vitamin A act in the lungs as antioxidants, trapping free radicals that can damage the lungs. Although such approaches may hold promise in controlled use, they can also pose potentially dangerous side effects and other consequences. Their focus on only one of the potential causes of cancer or emphysema may leave an individual unprotected from the effects of other potentially harmful substances. It is possible that the earliest fire-using hominid, *Homo erectus*, an individual of which died of hypervitaminosis A 1.6 million years ago east of Lake Turkana, Kenya, may have been attempting to dose himself with vitamin A–rich carnivore liver for its potential health benefits. He apparently overdosed on vitamin A, however, and died a rather painful death. Today chemotherapy, especially self-chemotherapy, can be just as dangerous and should be undertaken with due consultation with your physician (see chapter 14).

9

Diabetes Mellitus and the "Thrifty Genotype"

In the old days, physicians paid a lot of attention to a patient's urine—its amount, color, smell, and, believe it or not, its taste. If a person was producing a good deal of it, as if he or she was a siphon, the disease was called in Greek "diabetes" (Greek for "siphon"). If the urine smelled and tasted like honey, it was called "mellitus" (Greek for "honey"). The high levels of glucose found in a diabetic's bloodstream account for the overproduction of urine. The sugar molecules cause water to be pulled out of the cells as the body attempts to dilute the blood back to normal levels. This excess water is excreted by the kidney. Glucose can also spill over into the urine as the kidneys struggle to rid the body of the excess sugar, explaining its honeyed odor.

Today, diabetes mellitus affects some 16 million Americans and is the leading cause of adult blindness, kidney failure, and nontraumatic limb amputations. It kills more people each year than breast cancer. The most common form of diabetes, affecting 90 percent to 95 percent of diabetics, is termed "diabetes mellitus type II," or "non-insulin-dependent diabetes." This disease may go undiagnosed for years, and even when it is diagnosed it may be dismissed by many of its sufferers—until it is too late. It can lead to kidney failure, blindness, coma, gangrenous extremities, and, if left untreated, eventually death. It is still poorly understood by medical scientists. Medical textbooks frequently describe diabetes mellitus as a genetic and metabolic disease, but it actually begins as a normal metabolic reaction to an abnormal environment—one that we create within ourselves. Diabetes type II, which we discuss here, is a complicated disease,[1] but one that is made much more understandable from an evolutionary perspective.

Sugar Poisoning

The fundamental problem in diabetes is too much glucose in the blood. The sugar gets into your body in a pretty obvious way. You eat it—directly as sugar or in its complexed form as carbohydrate. Many people eat so much sugar that it becomes toxic, either directly causing damage to tissues, or indirectly hurting us by transforming itself into another harmful substance. For example, a derivative of glucose, sorbitol, can cloud the cornea of the eye, causing problems with vision. High sugar levels in our blood also cause cells to react in a way that is more than 2 billion years old.

Energy-rich glucose molecules have been primary food for living cells since the origin of cellular life. The orifice that liver and pancreatic beta cells employ for drinking in glucose is the "GLUT-2" (GLUT is short for "glucose transporter") receptor on the surface of the cell. Because glucose is normally rare in the environment, GLUT-2 receptors are ungated—that is, they let in any and all glucose molecules that come into contact with the cell membrane. Beta cells in the pancreas known as islets of Langerhans, which produce the hormone insulin (a Level 3 to 5 innovation), have many such GLUT-2 receptors. So do liver cells. This ever-open gateway for glucose is the fundamental etiology of diabetes mellitus.

With our high-sugar diets, we bathe our cells in glucose. The beta cells continue to function as they have for eons. They produce and release insulin into the bloodstream—and lots of it, because there is plenty of glucose. The liver cells continue to react as they have since ancient times—they happily imbibe the glucose, and use it or store it.

The second step in the development of diabetes now occurs. The insulin travels around the body until it reaches tissues that have orifices hungry for insulin—the insulin receptors found on skeletal muscle, heart muscle, and fat cells (collectively about two-thirds of a person's body weight). In these so-called peripheral cells, insulin acts like a key, opening a different receptor on the cell surface, GLUT-4, to let in glucose, essential for the cell's energy. But because there is now much more glucose flowing into the cell than the cell needs, it begins to transform itself. It reduces the number of insulin receptors on its surface. The flood of glucose entering the muscle or fat cell is thereby reduced to a more normal level. This reaction is what the muscle or fat cell has done since antiquity—regulate its internal environment to match energy needs with energy supply. But in a modern obese American's body, the peripheral cell's behavior sets into a motion a positive feedback loop that gives us diabetes if we continue to overload ourselves with a surfeit of glucose.

When the muscle and fat cells—which we now call "insulin resistant," because they have down-regulated their insulin receptors—cut off the inflow of glucose, it stays in the bloodstream. Glucose in the bloodstream increases and circulates back to the pancreatic beta cells, where it freely enters and initiates the production and release of even more insulin. The ever greater insulin levels continue to cause more and more insulin resistance in the muscle and fat tissues of the body, until finally almost no glucose can get into these cells. Most of the GLUT-4 receptors have been dismantled, and the cells begin to starve themselves.

This futile cycling finally takes its toll on the beta cells, and they begin to give out and die. The diabetic patient now has to rely on injections of insulin to maintain some supply of glucose to the muscle and fat cells.

Peripheral cells have simply tried to protect themselves from the extremely numerous insulin molecules by shutting them out—closing the cellular doors to the offending substance. Before single cells bonded together to create multicellular animal life-forms, they fended for themselves in the open sea by modifying the permeability of their cell walls. Molecules that they needed for sustained life and reproduction they allowed in; waste products and toxic molecules they attempted to extrude or prevent from entering.

We may ask why the beta cells in the pancreas do not have such a defensive mechanism against glucose. Why do the GLUT-2 receptors just stay open all the time, allowing glucose to flow into the cell? The GLUT-2 receptors date to a later phase of our evolution—when cells started living communally in large masses of cells called "organisms." Cells made compromises and lost some of their primitive characteristics as they became specialized for their new roles. GLUT-2 receptors are molecular adaptations of beta cells designed by evolution to transport glucose from the bloodstream to the cell when the concentration of glucose in the blood is higher than that of the cell. The beta cells gave up their primitive adaptation for self-protection in order to provide a signaling mechanism to the rest of the body for glucose availability. Mother Nature has bet that in most cases this adaptation will work well to deliver glucose to the cells when there is plenty of it around, usually just after we have eaten, so that it can be stored as fat or another energy storage molecule, glycogen. The system breaks down only when we upend the evolutionary applecart and overeat while expending very little energy.

Glucose and amino acids are the ultimate molecular components of what we eat. When cells in the small intestine detect food molecules, they release hormones into the blood that travel to the pancreas, where they stimulate the beta cells to release insulin into the blood. Insulin is the key that unlocks hungry cells and allows them to eat. Insulin travels around the body in the blood and "turns on" cells to drink in glucose and amino acids. Normally, glucose and amino acid levels in the blood are high just after we have eaten, and during this time insulin acts to move glucose and amino acids into cells, thus lowering blood levels of these substances. Insulin's effect is to make liver and fat cells turn glucose into storage molecules such as glycogen and fat, and to stimulate the making of protein from the amino acids.

Our cells also need sustenance when we have not eaten recently. When blood sugar is low, the alpha cells of the pancreas produce a "hormone of fasting" known as "glucagon." This hormone "turns off" muscle and fat cells to storing glucose and amino acids, and turns on liver cells to producing glucose, thus raising blood sugar.

Insulin and glucagon, normally acting in balanced opposition to each other, fail in their physiological role in diabetics primarily, as we have seen, because the receptor molecules for insulin on the body's cell membranes become drastically reduced in number. The diabetic's cells are deprived of glucose because their receptors are very reduced, and as the kidneys dump huge amounts of glucose from glucose-saturated blood, the body's cells are starving. Meanwhile, the body's high extracellular glucose and insulin levels are wreaking physiological havoc with the kidneys, the liver, the cardiovascular system, the eyes, and the nervous system. How could such a simple thing like too much sugar be so detrimental? We can only answer this question by looking at our evolutionary history.

Pleistocene Fat Storage and Diabetes

Two and a half million years ago, global climates shifted and the world began to plunge into a period of time colloquially called the Ice Age. Paradoxically, the Pleistocene was not only a time of seasonally quite cold temperatures, it also featured intervening periods of very warm temperatures. Cold temperatures became colder and warm temperatures became warmer. Seasons also became more marked within the cold and hot spells. In the highest latitudes, near the poles, glaciers and ice deposits were laid down, but in temperate and tropical regions, temperature fluctuations translated into extended droughts between the wet times.

What climate has to do with diabetes is that these changes affected the food sources of our ancestors, and our bodies evolved accordingly. When it rained there was plenty to eat, but when the rains stopped or the ice encroached, food became much scarcer. The fact that we are here today to contemplate these mysteries of the past proclaims that during our evolution as a species, not once did our direct ancestors fail to survive the challenges. Many of our ancestors' friends and relatives did not make it, however. Those of us who made it through the Pleistocene have fundamental adaptations to this fluctuating lifestyle that are still with us today.

We may characterize the Pleistocene lifestyle, not too inaccurately, as "feast or famine"—a balance between insulin and glucagon. When a fruiting tree was heavy with ripe fruit or the hunting group had bagged a mammoth, times were good. Human nature being what it is, most people didn't begin to worry about the next feast until their stomachs began growling. If the animals were around and the fruiting trees not too far away, they ate all they could hold. But if, because of circumstances beyond their control, no food was to be found other than a measly little root, tuber, or stray lizard, members of the group would begin to succumb to hunger, drop out of the daily trek, be picked off by predators, or otherwise be claimed by the grim reaper of natural selection. We know that many entire groups must have perished during the worst times of the Pleistocene, but somehow our ancestors survived. How?

The late James V. Neel, an anthropological geneticist at the University of Michigan, wrote a paper in 1962 in which he suggested that there was such a thing as a "thrifty genotype"—a particular genetic ability to turn ingested food quickly into fat, storing it for future times of famine.[2] Our bodies, in other words, would do what our conscious behavior did not or could not do—save for a rainless day. Neel suggested that the pancreas, the organ that lies nestled below our stomach,[3] became more rapidly responsive to an increase in the level of food molecules (blood sugar or glucose) in our bloodstream. Beta cells in the pancreas squirt out into the blood an "exciting" chemical—the hormone known as insulin[4]—that causes other cells in the body to suck up glucose, use it, and store it as fat or glycogen. Neel noted, "The individual whose pancreatic responses minimized post-prandial glycosuria[5] might have, during a period of starvation, an extra pound of adipose reserve." Not only that, Neel postulated that our ancestors were gluttonous. When the skinny ones had eaten their fill, our ancestors came back for seconds. If the pancreas continued to pump out insulin longer, sending glucose into storage, then blood sugar levels would still be low even after plenty of food had been eaten. The body's cells would still need glucose, we would still feel hungry, and thus we would continue to stuff our faces. Natural selection favored this piggish behavior because our more restrained friends and relatives just did not make it through the next big freeze-out between picnics.

Gluttons in the Land of Plenty

The thrifty genotype functioned well throughout the Pleistocene, but when modern civilization arose, things began to go awry. Our genetic and physiological mechanisms for smoothing out the hills and valleys of food availability were rendered redundant by our sophisticated agriculture, refrigeration, food processing, and distribution technologies. And our energy budgets changed drastically. We no longer have to run down game and carry heavy loads of foodstuffs miles back to camp. Nevertheless, we can do little about the ancient cravings that we have for lots of fat, salt, and sugar because our conscious mind just does not control our pancreas. Those cravings spelled survival and reproductive success for our ancestors. Because of that heritage, our bodies continue in our overfed civilization to store up energy reserves for a famine that never comes.

So what? Many people who have fought and lost the battle of the bulge have become resigned to their heroic proportions or Rubenesque figures. Even many physicians believe that adherence to a svelte body ideal is not necessarily optimal for health and that our pursuit of the thin can amount to a compulsion. But excess fat works significantly to the detriment of our physiology and ultimately our health. Diabetes is one of the very worst disease manifestations of obesity.

The thrifty genotype remains an important part of understanding diabetes, but parts of the hypothesis have had to be updated. Back in 1962, James Neel thought that obesity and diabetes were caused by an individual's increased secretion and release of insulin early in life. He thought that later on, the excess insulin caused an overproduction of another hormone from the pancreas, the "anti-insulin" that we now call glucagon.[6] Glucagon is produced by the alpha cells of the pancreas and generally counteracts the actions of insulin (produced by the beta cells), causing the liver to release glucose from glycogen storage molecules and thus raise blood glucose levels. Neel believed that long-standing overproduction of glucagon caused the high levels of blood glucose and somehow damaged the pancreas, causing glassy-looking ("hyalinized") areas under the microscope. We now know that this is not how diabetes develops. Glucagon disruption is not the basic cause of diabetes, as Neel supposed. Later researchers showed that "while glucagon may worsen the consequences of insulin lack, it is neither sufficient nor necessary for the development of diabetes."[7] Insulin and glucagon levels are disrupted in diabetes, but how did they get that way?

One of the missing keys to understanding the actions of insulin and glucagon was supplied by the discovery of receptor molecules imbedded in the cell membrane. One part sticks out of the cell. This part of the receptor binds to the hormone molecule. Another part extends from the cell membrane inside, projecting into the so-called cytosol, the internal watery environment of the cell. A circulating hormone in the blood is chemically recognized by the external part of the receptor molecule. The hormone binds to the receptor, docking like a small spacecraft to the mother ship, the cell. As soon as the hormone attaches, a "ground crew" of chemical messengers is sent out by the cell membrane, informing the cell that the hormone has arrived. Glucagon and insulin have different receptor molecules, and their actions comprise a coupled endocrine hormonal system. Glucagon, the fasting hormone, liberates stored glucose from glycogen and pushes the liver to produce glucose from amino acid precursors, keeping blood sugar high, while insulin, the "feasting hormone," opens the cellular gates to glucose and promotes its storage as glycogen and fat. This system maintains, under normal conditions, a balance in glucose supply to the body's cells.

In diabetes mellitus, the hormonal balance is lost. Experiments with animals provide our best estimates of how diabetes develops in human patients. A strain of lab rat known as the "Zucker diabetic fatty" shows a predictable progression of the disease when fed a high-sugar diet.[8] At first, the rats' pancreatic beta cells produce normal (high) amounts of insulin because there is a lot of glucose in the blood. Glucagon is virtually never secreted by the alpha cells because the rats never go without food, but the beta cells themselves attempt to regain an equilibrium of glucose levels. The beta cells act to slow down glycolysis, the process of breaking down glucose for energy, by reducing their secretion of the enzyme glucokinase, and to speed up gluconeogenesis, the process of building glycogen, by increasing their production of glucose-6-phosphatase, but all to no avail.

Because glucose keeps pouring in via the rat's diet, and the pancreas's beta cells are pumping out insulin at the maximum rate, the cells of the body continue to be bathed in insulin. And then, as we have seen, cells, particularly in the tissues that are insulin dependent for their glucose, such as resting muscles, begin to lose their insulin receptors. One hypothesis on how this happens is that receptor-molecular messenger complexes become degraded together within the cell (instead of the receptor releasing and migrating back to the cell membrane). This reduces the available pool of receptor molecules in the cell and ends up reducing the number of receptor sites on the cell's surface for binding insulin. This model explains how cells become "insulin insensitive" and let fewer glucose molecules into their interiors, causing blood glucose levels to soar.

In advanced diabetes mellitus, after starving cells have turned to alternative energy sources, using stored fat and muscle protein for energy, the overworked beta cells in the pancreas blink out and die. The term "hypoinsulinemic diabetes" is sometimes used to refer to this end stage of the disease, when insulin levels are low but glucose levels stay high. One widely accepted hypothesis is that the beta cells, working overtime, just wear out. Another idea is that the beta cells, because they are adapted to sensing glucose levels, lose any defense against toxic levels of glucose in the blood. Research on the gerbil *Psammomys obesus* shows that a high-calorie diet and high glucose levels in the blood lead to an initial increase in beta cell growth in the pancreas, but then kills off the beta cells. The authors of the study conclude that "glucotoxicity" is the reason.[9]

Neel's thrifty genotype hypothesis for the causation of diabetes mellitus thus been modified by newer research, but it still stands as an important heuristic explanation for the disease. Our ancestors did indeed evolve an effective adaptation to rapidly storing energy that could be used later. And that very efficiency is the root cause of diabetes that occurs when we have plenty of food for long periods of time.

Neel's hypothesis also helps to explain why certain groups of patients, such as African Americans and Native Americans, have higher rates of diabetes than Euro-Americans or Asian Americans.

Grains like wheat and rice have been dietary staples much longer in the Middle East and Eurasia than in most places in Africa and the Americas. Evolution has acted over the some 10,000 years of Eurasian human evolution to blunt the thrifty genotype, whereas only one to several generations in many African and Native American populations have been subjected to the high carbohydrate diets and glucotoxicity of Westernized diets. Physiological responses to excess glucose in such groups as the Pima Indians of New Mexico are magnified, and rates of diabetes are increased, because these populations have much more recently emerged from a hunter-gatherer lifestyle. The thrifty genotype hypothesis also has been used to explain the tendency toward obesity and diabetes among Polynesians, who, during their prehistoric colonization of vast regions of the Pacific, had to sustain long transoceanic voyages with little or no food resources.

In much the same way that a Formula One racecar never driven over 20 miles an hour runs very poorly, the body of a sedentary human being ceases to function well. Vigorous activity was a way of life for hunter-gatherers. Our bodies are evolved for hard work. Meriwether Lewis and William Clark, for example, observed a Native American traditional hunt in 1805 in which five men hauled out of a ravine numerous bison carcasses weighing a ton each for butchering. Tourists to rural Africa marvel at the weight that village women can carry on their backs. The skeletal remains of preagricultural peoples the world over show by their muscle markings that their level of strength and fitness vastly surpassed modern Westerners. It is little wonder then that diabetes was and still is an unknown disease among hunter-gatherers and other similarly active peoples.

Physical exercise increases the insulin sensitivity of muscle cells in the body, an adaptation that allows more glucose into these cells to perform work. Metabolic burning of glucose by the body's cells then decreases blood levels of glucose, which decreases the amount of insulin released by the beta cells of the pancreas and circulating in the bloodstream. All of these physiological effects disrupt the process of diabetes. From both evolutionary and physiological perspectives, we can now circumscribe the disease diabetes mellitus type II and clearly see how it can be brought under control.

Beating Diabetes

Mimicking our hunter-gatherer ancestors is the best way to cure diabetes. Number one on the list of behaviors to emulate is physical exercise. Physical exercise is a better way than any pharmaceutical agent available now or in the foreseeable future to return the pancreatic beta and alpha cells to their optimal, anciently evolved, functioning environments. By trial and error, physicians have also discovered that exercise, coupled with weight loss, is the most effective way to prevent diabetes and to ward off its symptoms once the disease has appeared.

Treating diabetes by behavioral modification is also the most reasonable treatment based on what we now know of the genetics of diabetes mellitus type II. A gene defect does not fundamentally cause diabetes. Rather, there are some genetic differences between and among human population groups that explain the varying degrees of the severity of the disease, but the disease itself is caused by chronic excess glucose in the bloodstream, obesity, and a lack of physical activity.

Physicians have also developed a "treatment of laziness" (perhaps a rather severe term) for those of their patients who will not or cannot follow a prescription of increased activity. All of the drugs employed in this modality of treatment are blunt instruments—they effect some benefits to the patient, but often with the cost of significant side effects. Four classes of oral diabetes drugs are now used. Sulfonylureas, such as tolbutamide and glimepiride, wring out of the already tired pancreatic beta cells the last dregs of insulin before they succumb to exhaustion, a process that usually takes about 10 years. They do this by blocking the ATP-sensitive potassium channels in the beta cells' membranes. Biguanides, such as metformin, override the liver's and the peripheral cells' resistance to insulin, but with the side effects of intestinal cramps, diarrhea, liver toxicity, and kidney toxicity. A third class of drugs, which includes Precose and miglitol, inhibit an intestinal enzyme, alpha-glucosidase, which keeps glucose from ever entering the bloodstream from the intestines. Flatulence, from gas released by bacterial decay of the undigested food in the colon, is a major side effect. A fourth category of drug, the thiazolidinediones, includes Rezulin, which was taken off the market in March 2000 because of over 60 deaths from liver failure associated with its use. The mode of action of these drugs is to resensitize liver cells to insulin. Newer drugs in the same class, Actos and Avandia, have replaced Rezulin. Side effects of these drugs mostly relate to hepatotoxicity—damage and death to liver cells.

Even with intensive use of the battery of antidiabetic pharmaceuticals, more than 50 percent of sufferers from diabetes mellitus type II have poor control of their blood glucose, and, according to one study, some 18 percent of these patients develop serious medical complications within six years of diagnosis.[10] But the drugs are effective, at least for a while, for many patients who by choice or necessity do not change to a more evolutionarily centric lifestyle. These people are living on borrowed time, hoping against hope that their beleaguered and drugged cells will hold out a little longer. Behavioral change—becoming physically active and eating a balanced diet low in calories—is the best prescription for diabetics. A responsible pharmaceutical regime that helps a diabetic patient take an active role in his or her own recovery from the disease by exercising and eating well has an important role in treatment. The pharmaceutical treatment of laziness is associated with significant and even life-threatening side effects, and it cannot come close to the therapeutic success of the Paleolithic prescription. Physicians should prescribe it cautiously, and patients concerned with their own health can do much better.

10

Gout, Liver Enzymes, and Global Climate Change

In the past, a certain celebrity was attached to having gout because the disease was considered a malady of the wealthy, of the epicure and the bon vivant, afflicting such personages as Benjamin Franklin and Samuel Johnson. Today, however, it affects some 9 million Americans every year, and is recognized for what it is—an inflammation of the joints with associated kidney problems.

The medical textbooks classify gout as a "metabolic disease," implying that something has gone awry in our enzyme systems to raise the levels of the metabolite uric acid so high that urate crystals become lodged in the joints, causing terrible pain. This is not strictly correct. *Everyone* in the species *Homo sapiens* lacks the enzyme, urate oxidase, which is necessary to degrade urate (the sodium-complexed salt of uric acid found in the blood) into its harmless product, allantoin. Unlike urate, allantoin is very water soluble and easily excreted in urine. Scientists have tried for some time to relate urate to human evolution—just as they have tried to determine why we lack this enzyme, when almost all other primates and mammals have it—but until recently we did not have enough information to come to any reasonable conclusion. Now we do.

Urate, Big Brains, and Gout

In 1955 a geophysical engineer at MIT named Egon Orowan published a paper in the British science journal *Nature* entitled "The Origin of Man." This event—an engineer publishing an article on human evolution in a major journal—would be worthy of note in itself, but Orowan's message was equally unusual. He proposed that higher primate intellectual ability owed its evolutionary impetus to the lack of a liver enzyme. Known as urate oxidase, or uricase for short, it breaks down urate, a known brain stimulant, in the body. Orowan's "brain hypothesis" of urate evolution maintained that the consequent buildup in the bloodstream of urate accounts for the increased intellectual abilities of the great apes and man.

Of course, the downside of a high level of urate in the body is that it causes gout. Could gout really be caused by an adaptation ultimately related to large brain size and increased intellectual ability—attributes that we consider uniquely human?

Strangely, gout afflicts Western and industrialized societies much more than Third World or hunter-gatherer cultures. This is not what one would expect for an adaptation that should be specieswide. Orowan had an answer for this observation. Urate is formed in the body by the breakdown of purines, which are in high concentrations in meat. People in the industrialized countries eat much more meat, and Orowan thought that they may do this in order to stimulate their brains with high urate levels. Orowan also posits a role for urate in causing what he calls "pressure-of-life" diseases, because "this stimulant can be a more powerful inhibitor of rest and recovery from work [than caffeine or theobromine]."[1]

Scientists largely ignored Orowan's brain hypothesis, not only because it was opposed by one of the great evolutionary biologists of the day, J. B. S. Haldane, but also because many physical anthropologists at the time were not trained in and did not appreciate biochemistry. Urate oxidase deficiency to them might just as well have been pure gibberish. Today, most experts on human evolution call themselves "biological anthropologists" and practice a much more interdisciplinary approach. But Orowan's short paper of over 40 years ago has been virtually forgotten. How do we test his intriguing idea?

A Comparative Approach to Testing the Brain Hypothesis

Hypotheses in evolutionary biology are complex constructions, requiring a combination of both history and the experimental method. But because immense amounts of time are required for evolution to work, and because we cannot manipulate long stretches of time in the laboratory, we must look for natural experiments that have already taken place. Charles Darwin pioneered this comparative approach, and today's evolutionary scientists, be they molecular biologists, paleontologists, or anthropologists, still use it in testing their hypotheses.

In looking at the comparative biochemistry of urate metabolism across the animal kingdom, we find that most animals break down the purines in their food to uric acid, and then on to the relatively innocuous and water-soluble compound called allantoin, and finally to urea. Urea is voided with excess water in the urine. This biochemical chain of reactions, known as "purine catabolism," is one of the very important ways that the body prevents a buildup of toxic ammonia in the body; think of the strong ammonia smell of a pail of wet baby diapers, courtesy of bacterial degradation. Fish, amphibians, and almost all mammals share this primitive biochemical pathway. But some animals—insects, snails, reptiles, birds, and a few scattered mammals—lack the enzymes necessary to degrade purines any further than uric acid. Because these hodgepodge creatures are not closely related, their shared characteristic of "uricosuria" (uric-acid-containing urine, which in turn is indicative of high blood levels of uric acid) must be independently evolved. We know that the ancestors of the uricosuric animals were able to break down purines all the way to allantoin and urea. So we must deduce that the genetic mutations that altered the normal biochemistry in these populations of animals had to have arisen independently of one another, and had to have been advantageous, each in its own right, in promoting the survival and reproduction of the species.

Comparing the various species that have lost the ability to break down uric acid, with a view towards assessing the likelihood of Orowan's hypothesis, we are immediately struck with the fact that the vast majority of the brainiest animals, the mammals, do not have high blood levels of urate. And those animals that do, with very few exceptions (such as ourselves), are not known for their intellectual prowess.

Orowan's hypothesis also suffers when we look at people who have abnormally high blood levels of urate, a medical condition known as "hyperuricemia." Hyperuricemia predisposes individuals to develop gout, especially in the big toe. Do these patients show the increased brain stimulation posited by Orowan? Are they more stressed? Do they suffer from insomnia, as we might suspect from the postulated physiological effects of uric acid? A review of the clinical literature fails to reveal any of these characteristics or symptoms, as generally reported by gout sufferers (except that the pain in their toes can clearly be a major cause for stress and can even keep them up at night). It appears that Orowan's is one of those beautiful hypotheses slain by ugly facts, to paraphrase Thomas Henry Huxley.

Free Radicals Sopped up by Urate

Biochemists next became interested in the evolutionary biology of uric acid and urate. Twenty-six years after Orowan's paper, bio-chemist Bruce Ames of the University of California, Berkeley, and colleagues proposed an "antioxidant hypothesis." They suggested that the inability of humans and a few other animals to break down uric acid was an adaptation to reduce internal damage to the membranes and DNA of the body's cells caused by the action of oxygen free radicals.[2] These species of atoms lack one or more orbiting electrons in their outer shells and are consequently prone to react with other atoms, stealing electrons from them and in turn converting them into free radicals. Free radicals are formed in the body by a number of processes, but oxygen metabolism in the cells and skin exposure to sunlight are thought to be the two major sources of these damaging particles, at least in nonsmokers. Free radicals have been implicated in the aging process, in cancer, and in many degenerative diseases.

Ames proposed to add urate to the list of the body's defenses and repair mechanisms to deal with the challenge posed by free radicals. Our diet has a lot to do with helping us cope. Linus Pauling's famous prescription for massive doses of vitamin C had its biochemical basis in the prevention of free radical damage. Vitamins A and E are also active in the biochemical conversion of free radicals to less harmful species of the oxygen atom. Ames pointed out that the molecular structure of uric acid can act in this capacity, but at issue is whether at normal human physiological concentrations and in life it does act this way.

Ames's supporters point out that in primates, species with high levels of urate live longer in general. But in actuality, this is only a two-point correlation—all monkeys and "lower" primates, the prosimians, can break down uric acid (like most other mammals), but apes and humans as a group cannot. There is no progressive increase in urate levels as primate life spans increase. Life spans in primates primarily vary as functions of metabolic rate and of body size. Smaller species with high heart rates and cell turnover rates die sooner than larger primates. Plotting urate levels and life spans of a few apes and other smaller primates does show a weak correlation, but this is purely by chance. The correlation is a reflection of other evolutionary events—that apes and humans are the largest of the primates and have therefore the slowest metabolisms.

Another test of Ames's hypothesis is to look at human patients with hyperuricemia and gout. Do they show any beneficial effects of their high uric acid levels? Clinical reports show the opposite, in fact. Gout patients have higher chances of developing a large number of cancers, including leukemias, colon cancer, and rare joint carcinomas. Equally, there is no evidence that individuals with high urate levels or gout live longer or have any protection from disease because of the supposed antioxidant effects of uric acid. As in the case of the brain hypothesis, the antioxidant hypothesis for urate is not supported by either evolutionary evidence or by clinical results.

Savannas, Water Conservation, and Uric Acid

In comparing uricosuric species (like ourselves) with urea- and allantoin-excreting species, one primary environmental characteristic stands out. Uricosuric species are virtually all adapted to dry terrestrial habitats in which water conservation is at a premium.

Land-living snails and insects excrete uric acid, unlike their aquatic ancestors. Reptiles evolved a leathery egg that can be laid on land and a tough, dry skin that is not subject to drying out. Birds similarly lay shelled eggs on land and then take to the air, although some species have become secondarily adapted to a water-tied existence. And among the mammals, the desert-living gerbils, the Dalmatian coach hound (bred for extended running in the hot, dry environment of the Balkan coast),[3] and, curiously, human beings and apes all share this characteristic. Uricosuria must be related to conserving water.

The large amount of water required to excrete urea in most animals provides a solution as to why uricosuria would be an advantageous adaptation. Some water is saved by truncating the biochemical degradation of uric acid to allantoin, since two molecules of water are required for every molecule of uric acid degraded, and then in the next step, two more molecules of water are required to reduce a molecule of allantoin to a urea molecule. But the real value of excreting the relatively insoluble uric acid is that significant water can be reabsorbed by the kidney. For animals living in an environment with plenty of water, reducing the relatively reactive and potentially gout-causing uric acid molecules to the inert urea molecules makes physiological sense, and evolution has consequently smiled on this adaptation for these species. But such a lavish use of water molecules to flush out urea by animals in more arid environments leads to a thirsty death. The grim reaper of natural selection only lets pass those individuals in a population with mutations that can conserve water.

This scenario makes sense for such animals as lizards, birds, gerbils, and Dalmatians, but how can it be true for the apes and humans? Apes are well known denizens of dense tropical forests, and humans need to drink water at least daily, especially in hot and dry climates. At first this observation seems damning to our hypothesis, but a view of the fossil record makes it much more plausible.

In the middle part of the Miocene epoch, some 17 to 12 million years ago, as evidenced by fossil sites in Africa and indeed the world over, there was a global shift to drier conditions.[4] Grasslands spread and forests shrank. The equatorial forest belt that extended from the Atlantic to the Indian Oceans in Africa broke up into patches, particularly on the eastern side of the continent around the Great Rift Valley. Great swaths of Eurasian forests disappeared as the Himalayas rose up, blocked rain clouds, and changed climate patterns. Grazing and browsing herbivores, which had the high-crowned molar teeth indicating adaptations to open-country conditions, appeared in large numbers. Apes great and small, which up to this point in time had lived in swarms in the forests, now went extinct in droves. Only a few of the apes survived, adapting to the drier conditions outside the forests by evolving thick molar tooth enamel to cope with the tougher foods, or by staying small and holding their own within patches of the forest that remained. The first group of survivors consisted of relatively large woodland apes that we have come to know by the names *Kenyapithecus*, *Equatorius*, *Afropithecus*, and *Turkanapithecus* in Africa,[5] and by the names *Sivapithecus* and *Ouranopithecus* in Eurasia.[6] The second group of small forest apes is largely hypothetical because we know of them only by deduction from molecular evolutionary evidence derived from living species and by circumstantial paleontological evidence.[7] But they are of interest to us because they include our ancestors.

The Miocene woodland apes eventually all died out, because things just got worse in the late Miocene, between 12 and 5 million years ago. Climates continued to become drier and woodlands devolved into savannas, or plains, some nearly treeless. In retrospect, these species in the game of natural selection had made their move out of the forests too early, and they were caught between the proverbial evolutionary rock and climatic hard place. They paid the price of extinction, by the reckoning of most anthropologists. But the second group had more evolutionary room in which to maneuver—they were forest dwellers who had another shot at making it when even their forest patches began to dwindle. And we now know they had biomolecular adaptations that allowed them to conserve water.

Sometime in the latter part of the Miocene, the ancestors of the gibbon, the "lesser" ape that lives today in Southeast Asia, underwent a mutation that truncated the metabolic pathway of uric acid to urea, disrupting the function of the enzyme urate oxidase. This adaptation is perhaps the most eloquent evidence yet that the gibbon went through a period of degradation of its forest habitat. The species is today an obligate forest dweller swinging from trees in feats of acrobatic virtuosity. The mutation that the gibbon underwent was a deleted length of 13 base pairs of DNA between codons 72 and 76 (a codon is the three-letter nucleotide code in DNA specifying a specific amino acid) within the gene that codes for the enzyme urate oxidase.[8] This deletion disrupted the function of the gene and results in the gibbon, like people, having no ability to degrade uric acid to urea.

The common ancestor of hominids (ourselves) and the "great" apes (chimp, gorilla, and orang), which we know by fossil evidence had diverged from the lineage of the gibbon by the middle of the Miocene epoch (about 15 million years ago), also underwent mutational change that disrupted the function of urate oxidase. But in a fascinating twist, the gene mutation in the hominid–great ape lineage was a different one from that of the gibbon—a nonsense mutation at codon 33 of the gene. The mutation had occurred at close to the same time (15 million years ago) as the mutation in the same gene in the gibbon, but at a different place in the gene and in a different way. The conclusion from this surprising finding is that the water-saving uricosuria adaptation of the great apes and humans was an independent evolutionary event from the water-saving uricosuria adaptation of the gibbon. Selection for conserving water must have been severe, and the latter part of the Miocene epoch undoubtedly saw the deaths of large numbers of thirsty apes who could not make the trek from one patch of life-sustaining forest to another. These ancient, epic life-and-death struggles of our ape forebears have been masked until now because apes surviving into the modern world have retired back into the forests as their primary adaptive homes. Only humans ventured farther out, into the savannas, where we find their fossils in the succeeding Pliocene epoch, beginning 5 million years ago.

For our hominid ancestors, the urate oxidase gene mutation served an important function, allowing them to disperse across relatively arid terrain with little surface water. It likely also played a role in the evolution in the hominids of a sweat-cooled, largely hairless body, a use for the conserved metabolic water not elaborated by any of the other ape lineages. But for most humans in the modern world, the inability to break down urate in the body is nothing more than evolutionary baggage. The mutation only comes back to haunt us in the form of the disease called gout.

Treating Gout

From a clinical standpoint, slightly higher levels of urate in the body pose no problem. But for an overfed and sedentary few, urate levels become excessively high, and they develop gout, a painful form of arthritis in which crystals form in the joints. Dining to excess regularly on foods rich in purines, which are metabolized into urate, will elevate urate levels tremendously. And if these epicures do not regularly exercise, their bodies will not use the excess purines to make new muscle and connective tissue, and urate will continue to build up.

When urate levels get high enough, crystals of sodium urate form in the body. They may be found in the kidneys as renal stones and in the skin as yellowish white "tophi," but when they reside in the joints, doctors diagnose the condition as gout. The joint between the first metatarsal bone in our feet and the first phalanx of our big toe is the most common place gout sufferers complain about, probably because this joint bears a great deal of weight and causes sheer agony when the sufferer walks.

The excruciating pain gout sufferers experience, coupled with their usually relatively high socioeconomic statuses, has led to an inordinate amount of medical attention having been paid to gout over the years. Rheumatologists, physicians who specialize in joint diseases, prescribe treatments based on prevailing theories about what causes the disease. Until recently, most rheumatologists believed that gout was solely a metabolic disease, similar to a rare and inborn inability to synthesize another enzyme important in purine metabolism, HGPRT,[9] and a disease that also increases levels of uric acid. HGPRT enzyme deficiency leads to Lesch-Nyhan syndrome, and the increase in urate in the body results from a blockage of the normal pathway. The disease causes significant neurological dysfunction, particularly self-mutilation, in the children that are affected. But gout is different. There is no specific enzymatic deficiency in the people who suffer from gout—all members of the species lack the enzyme. The explanation for the disease then should rest not on a biochemical characteristic that we all have, but rather on the differential behavioral, dietary, or environmental histories that gout sufferers present.

The long-term, "adaptive normality" cure for gout is to eat a low-purine diet (Table 6), stop drinking alcohol in any more than moderate amounts, and begin regular and normal exercising. But failing that (and most gout patients do fail at this), is there a more immediate therapy that our evolutionary scenario suggests for this disease?

The traditional therapy for gout is a medicine called "colchicine." This is a chemical that is also used in studies of chromosomes because it disables the little spindle fibers that pull the chromosomes apart to the opposite sides in a dividing cell. It is sometimes called a "mitotic poison" because it stops the process of cell division ("mitosis"). This blunt instrument medicine does not sound like a good substance to ingest, but like so much in the trial-and-error business of allopathic medicine, it has been found to work. Gout sufferers report remarkable improvement and relief from pain. Colchicine apparently inhibits the inflammatory response of macrophages and monocytes, thus reducing the amounts of substance P and other pain-causing agents released, but there are also side effects. Other rapidly dividing cells, particularly those in the

Table 6. Purine Content of Some Foods

Gout sufferers should avoid foods with high purine levels.

Foods with Very High Purine Levels:	Foods with High Purine Levels:
Anchovies, brains, gravies, kidneys, sardines, sweetbreads	Bacon, beef, calf tongue, carp, chicken soup, codfish, duck, goose, halibut, lentils, perch, pork, rabbit, sheep, shellfish, trout, turkey, veal, venison

Foods with Moderately High Purine Levels:	Foods with Low Purine Levels:
Asparagus, bluefish, bouillon, cauliflower, chicken, crab, ham, herring, kidney beans, lima beans, lobster, mushrooms	Navy beans, oatmeal, oysters, peas, salmon, spinach, tripe, tuna

Source: MotherNature.com Health Encyclopedia, Portland, Oregon

gut, are also inhibited, and significant gastric and intestinal distress can result. Extensive use can result in low red and white blood cell counts, anemia, and reduced immune function.

An alternative pharmacological treatment, now that the "defect" can be genetically pinpointed, is to replace the single gene product—in this case, urate oxidase. With new recombinant genetic technologies, urate oxidase can now be produced efficiently and made available to gout sufferers. Recent clinical results are very promising for this replacement of a gene product missing from the human constitution for about 15 million years. Not only is synthetic urate oxidase more reasonable as a treatment for gout from the standpoint of evolutionary medicine, it may also be much less expensive for the patient.

Gout is rarely a life-threatening disease, but it is a good example of a modern disease with evolutionary roots in our hominoid (Level 14) ancestry. In the next chapter we turn to ailments whose origins are to be found in the successive, hominid stage of our evolution.

11

Back Pain, Bad Knees, and Flatfeet

Because our brains can conceive remarkable feats and activities, and because human anatomy is generalized and in a sense multipurpose, we humans tend to forget our bodies have their limits. This has undoubtedly been of great natural-selective value in the human past. We might well imagine exhausted hunters pushing onward to bag a wounded mammoth, which then feeds the entire tribe in winter, or a parent who carries an injured or sick child, unable to walk, on a long trek when the group has to move. Such heroic feats could and did spell the difference between survival and death. The heavy muscle markings and the frequent trauma-induced osteoarthritis on our ancestors' fossil bones document their hard, physical lives—and the realities of our musculoskeletal system.

We are apelike primates who only recently adopted bipedality, evolved large body size, and expanded our behavioral capabilities to a tremendously wide range of activities.[1] Today, many of these activities, such as pushing pencils and shuffling papers, don't require us to keep in shape. If we are to avoid injury and pain to our

147

musculoskeletal system, we must be aware of our body's evolved capabilities and adjust our activities around our central zone of adaptation. This chapter is about modern human orthopedic ailments—how to understand them in evolutionary context and how to prevent them.

Orthopedic Evolution

The term "orthopedics"—meaning "straight foot"—belies our anthropocentric bias in dealing with medical problems of our muscular and skeletal systems. The term goes back to a time when surgeons treated clubfoot, a birth defect in which an infant's foot curled in like an ape's. Orthopedic medicine later expanded to include treatment of any other parts of the body that were not "straight," that is, correctly aligned in a vertical plane when we stand up straight. But this assumption, that uprightness is intrinsic to the human condition, is wrong.

Many aspects of our bodies are designed for a life on all fours or, alternatively, a life in the trees. As we saw in chapter 2, bipedalism is a relatively recent evolutionary acquisition for hominids—only some 5 million years old on present evidence. In contrast, running adaptations in the horse lineage are some 40 million years old, and swimming among sea mammals goes back about 55 million years. Nevertheless, walking and running work well for most humans, but there are many caveats to this rather precarious way of moving around.

Evolution stacked our vertebrae to balance our large, globular head and upper body on our legs. The vertebral column normally sags in four places—two facing forward (in our neck and lower back) and two facing backward (in our upper back and pelvic region). Our close relatives, the great apes, have none of this sagging.[2] Their vertebral columns describe smooth, slight, backward curves from their skull to their pelvis, very much like a suspension bridge, nicely supported by contact with the ground of the arms in front and legs behind.

When one examines the individual bones of an ape spine and compares them with those in humans, there are surprisingly few anatomical adaptations that separate the two—remarkable when we think of how centrally important bipedalism is for human beings, but understandable when we consider how relatively recent our upright adaptation is. Ligaments, cartilage, and muscles attaching to our apelike vertebral column—not the bones themselves— provide the primary support for the spinal curves of bipedalism in our moving and living bodies.

Human limbs also evolved in concert with the novel hominid way of walking. Human arms, no longer involved in moving the body around, are shorter, but otherwise they are very similar to the arms of the great apes. In contrast, the human pelvis and lower limbs are radically different. They have evolved to bear all the weight of the body and provide the rigid support to the muscles propelling us forward when we walk and run. The pelvis, connecting the legs to the spinal column, thus has become a wide, shallow, and more heavily built structure in hominids than in apes. The legs have lengthened to increase stride and have straightened to facilitate balance and the vertical transfer of our body weight to the ground.

Our feet are the most changed from our ape ancestral condition. They have transformed from dual-function organs that supported half the body's weight on the outside and grasped with a thumblike big toe on the inside, to become stiff supporting arches balancing all the body's weight above them.[3] Our feet reflect, more than any other part of our body, the change from a life in the trees to one on the ground. But like the spine, these changes in the human foot have happened quickly, and we retain in our feet many reminders of our arboreal heritage. From an evolutionary standpoint, we would expect problems from such an unusual and recently developed anatomy, and indeed we have them.

Back Pain

One recent study estimated that 80 percent of Americans have had back pain sufficiently severe at some time in their lives to visit a doctor or seek treatment. Back pain by this and other estimates is the single most common ailment of modern people, accounting for more lost days of work than any other single cause except the common cold. In a smaller number of people, back pain is a chronic condition, seriously affecting quality of life and limiting activities. In a significant subset of back pain sufferers, the pain is acute—so bad that it is debilitating and immobilizing.

Compared to the magnitude of the problem, there is precious little that a doctor can do to alleviate your back pain. Painkillers are usually only partially effective, and they have so many negative side effects, such as drowsiness and nausea, that some patients feel that they are worse off for the treatment. Surgery has not proved an effective solution for chronic back pain, either, except in cases in which there is a discrete injury to the spine or vertebrae that can be corrected. But even in cases of "slipped disk"—when a joint between vertebrae breaks down and the spinal nerves emerging from the spinal cord are compressed—10-year follow-up studies show that patients who had surgery have fared about the same as those who did not. Spinal manipulation, as practiced by chiropractors, and massage can relax your back, but they provide only temporary relief for chronic back pain. There are no genes that explain back pain. There are no back-pain-causing infectious agents that can be counteracted with immunizations or antibiotics. Where do we look for a medical solution? A good place to start is human anatomy, the most basic of the medical sciences.

The anatomical pattern of sensory nerve branches to the spine, to its ligaments, and to its muscles in large part explains where chronic back pain comes from. Pain receptors are nerve endings that detect tissue damage, too much stretch, too much pressure, or lack of oxygen and blood supply to the tissue. They are liberally scattered in the surface of vertebrae, but not inside them. So the back pain from a collapsing vertebra in old-age osteoporosis comes not from the inside of the crumbling bone, but from its surface.

The ligaments holding vertebrae together are also copiously supplied with sensitive nerve endings. If ligaments become inflexible and tight from lack of normal activity and then are wrenched by sudden flexing, extending, or rotation, they can tear, causing exquisite pain. The damage can be microscopic in scale but loom large in our consciousness.

Muscular tension or spasm is also a major contributor to back pain. Because of our incomplete skeletal and ligamentous adaptations to upright posture, muscular action helps to sustain our spinal curvatures. If our normal muscular strength is not maintained, the remaining muscles in our backs are overworked as they attempt to maintain our vertical vertebral column. Many working postures, such as sitting slouched at a keyboard, produce a significant amount of muscle fatigue and can contribute to back pain.

Bipedalism also predisposes our spines to very painful displacement of vertebrae—the fearsome slipped disk. In fact, this orthopedic problem is caused by a tearing of the ring of fibrous connective tissue that sits atop a vertebra, allowing the semiliquid center of the intervertebral disk (nucleus pulposus) to ooze out. The pain does not come from either the tear or the oozing out of the nucleus pulposus because there seem to be few or no pain-transmitting nerves in either place. Rather, the protrusion presses directly on a spinal nerve as the nerve leaves the spinal cord between vertebrae. This is the reason that a slipped disk not only hurts in your back, but also frequently radiates pain into your legs, which the lower spinal nerves also supply. The injury to an intervertebral disk usually happens when we are flexing our vertebral column—that is, bending over. Excessive weight, from lifting or from our own body weight, dislocates a vertebra forward, tearing the back part or outside ring of the disk, the annulus fibrosus. Compared to most ligament- and muscle-derived back pain, the pain of a herniated disk is excruciating. What can evolutionary medicine offer in way of a solution?

The Ape's Solution to Back Pain

Despite the fact that our backs are not "perfect" adaptations from an engineering standpoint, human hunter-gatherers do not suffer from chronic back pain. Neither, apparently, do the free-ranging apes have chronic back problems. Examining how our lives differ from these baseline conditions provides an evolutionary perspective on back pain and how to alleviate it.

Many people who have chronic back pain ascribe their symptoms to a "bad bed." How do apes sleep in order to avoid back problems? Michael Tetley examined ape and primitive human sleeping patterns from a standpoint of normal musculoskeletal function.[4] Apes make simple "nests" of vegetation on the ground, similar to simple beds of humans, but both are hard, being in direct contact with the ground, and lack "pillows." Living nonhuman hominoids most commonly sleep on their sides, with the supporting shoulder hunched to make a straight line from the side of the body to the neck and the head. Sometimes the arm is flexed and used as a support for the head. Interpolating between modern apes and modern, technologically primitive humans, it is probable that australopithecines slept the same way. Until recently, the modern Western ideal for a place to sleep was softness, cushiness, and plushness. But a soft substrate on which to sleep also means a bent spinal column, stress on vertebral ligaments, and tensed muscles all night to prevent hyperextension or hyperflexion of joints. A very firm mattress is the best compromise.

Apes do not carry things for long distances. Experiments in which Jane Goodall provided free-ranging chimps with too many bananas showed that these apes will attempt to carry food in their hands for short distances while walking on two legs. But they cannot keep this up for long. The muscle fatigue from their extensor back muscles finally gets to be too much, and they fall forward onto their knuckles, dropping whatever it was that they were carrying.

Human carrying behavior is different. Humans are, of course, habitually bipedal, and carrying behavior is almost certainly ancient (Level 15). People do carry things long distances, but the burdens cannot be too heavy, and it is best to carry them aligned with our vertebral column. In a place like East Africa, where beasts of burden are relatively rare, traditional people still carry most of what they want to move from one place to another. A Western visitor cannot fail to be struck at how massive the loads are that are carried by slight African women walking along the rural roadside. Loads are either balanced on the head or carried on the back, supported by straps from the forehead. Heavy loads are never carried out in front, as Westerners would generally attempt to do.

The Western manner of picking up and carrying heavy loads— in the front—accounts for a large number of back injuries. The spine is flexed, the intervertebral disks are stressed, especially in the back, and tears in the ligaments occur. Paradoxically, weakness in the abdominal muscles on the front of our bodies also contributes to a lessening of support for our back because we cannot sustain the increased abdominal pressure helping to push the body upright. In preventing lifting injuries to the back, it certainly helps to pick up loads from a squatting position and then use our legs to rise to a standing position. But it is safer and less fatiguing to carry heavy loads on our back, over our shoulder, or, if we can attain the necessary skill, balanced on our heads.

Soft beds and improper lifting explain a large number of cases of back pain. But many Americans who have firm beds and never lift anything heavier than a bag of groceries have chronic back pain. What explains their pain? Again, free-ranging apes and aboriginal hominids suggest an answer. Like all animals, we hominids evolved to lead active lives. Our muscles were exercised and well developed, our joints were actively moved and lubricated on a daily basis, and the amount of stored fat in our body was low. The average, inactive, modern American has poor muscle tone, stiff joints, and far too much body fat (mostly on the front of his or her body). Even without picking up anything in your hands, a tremendous amount of stress is placed on your vertebral column. A poorly developed musculoskeletal system can do little to counteract the increased burden. The modern epidemic in back pain is a side effect of the modern epidemic in obesity.

Origins of Hip, Knee, and Foot Bony Ailments

As we saw in chapter 2, the hominid pelvis changed substantially through evolution—from a narrow, elongated, apelike pattern to a wide-hipped and thick structure with a very strong hip joint. We generally have few problems with our hips dislocating, although problems may develop when the bone itself begins to deteriorate in old age (osteoporosis). We do have major problems with our knees coming undone. Operations to repair injured knee tissues are the most common (and most profitable) procedure performed by orthopedic surgeons in America. And while our feet do not generally dislocate, many of us do have problems with sprained ankles, flatfeet, bunions, and chronic foot pain. Feet are so much trouble to Americans that specialty medical practitioners known as "podiatrists," who have dedicated professional schools and separate professional degrees, have developed to treat them. This variable but widespread pattern of ailments in our lower limbs is a challenge to understanding, but a comparative and evolutionary perspective assists us.

The hip joint in apes functions similarly to the hominid hip joint. Apes support their bodies more or less vertically at the hip joint, although sometimes the thigh may be stretched out at an angle that makes all of us—except ballet dancers—wince. The ape knee, on the other hand, is a rotational joint, allowing the lower leg to rotate around the thigh for the purpose of gaining a foothold on a convenient branch. We conceive of the human knee as a "hinge" joint, but in fact it is a flat, apelike (and potentially mobile) joint held in place only by a few cartilages, ligaments, and muscle tendons. When a football tackle attempts to realign another player's knee into the old apelike posture, these tissues can be rent. Most knee injuries occur on the inside of the knee, because the lateral side of the knee in our ape ancestors had stronger ligaments to support the weight of the body against gravity.

The human foot is a structure that bears many reminders of our climbing heritage. Podiatrists and orthopedists may think that the ideal "straight" posture of the foot is from the heel to the ball of the foot—and in strict bipedal walking, they are correct. But the true anatomical axis of the human foot is oriented long the lines of the ancient ape foot, adapted for grasping large branches between the big toe and the second toe. The ape foot axis runs from these toes back, not to the heel, but to the outside of the ankle, where body weight was supported while holding onto a vertical tree branch. Our longitudinal foot arch, so long considered a well-designed, bridgelike structure uniquely designed for bipedalism, is really an incurved part of our foot originally designed to caress the roundness of trees.

With this perspective on the foot's evolved anatomy, most modern ailments of the foot can be understood.[5] A "flatfoot" results when excessive body weight, combined with poor muscle tone, collapses the longitudinal arch. Our ankle-flexing muscles, which loop up under the arch, attempt to hold the bones up, but in this they are doomed to failure. Leg and foot pain result. If foot joints, like the big toe or the midtarsal joint, are mobile like an ape's—genetic variations about which we can do little—we have the same problem. Muscle-strengthening exercises, a normal body weight, and supporting orthotic arch supports for the weak or movable joints can allow a person to walk and even run without pain.

Varicose Veins and Hemorrhoids

Maladies of a different variety affect our lower limbs because we are bipeds. The veins of our body are thin-walled blood vessels with relatively low blood pressure. The heart pushes blood through our arteries at high pressure, and when the blood emerges from our capillaries to enter the veins for the return trip to our lungs and heart, its flow is slower. The arteries have encircling smooth muscle coverings that squeeze blood through the vessels when they contract. The veins mostly lack smooth muscle. The skeletal muscles in our limbs, contracting as we move about, play an important role in pressing blood out of the veins and back to our heart. So if we are inactive for long periods, the lower parts of our bodies—our legs if we are standing, or our pelvic veins if we are sitting—collect venous blood.

Veins in our limbs have an adaptation that acts to prevent backflow of blood. Small one-way valves let blood through only in the direction back to the heart. But if there is little or no muscle contraction to push the blood along, it builds up against the closed valves, distending the veins. These distended parts of veins are termed "varicosities," and if they become large they can become painful and inflamed. Chronically inflamed varicose veins in our legs lead to a debilitating condition known as "phlebitis," which is potentially life threatening if a blood clot breaks off and lodges in another part of our body, such as the lungs. Phlebitis is a hominid-only malady to which we are predisposed by our upright posture. In our aboriginal mode of life, which featured plenty of walking, running, and carrying, blood was pushed back to the heart through the passive squeezing of our skeletal muscles. But with a life of inactivity or an occupation that requires standing in one place for long periods of time, blood that is not squeezed back to the heart collects in our legs, resulting in the tortuous distensions of varicose veins. Surgery is an imperfect solution of last resort because it rarely completely solves the problem, especially if the initiating factors are not resolved. As prevention, in addition to exercising, we can alleviate most of the problem if we raise our legs when we can to drain the blood back to our heart, or wear wear elastic stockings to help venous blood return from our legs.

A similar condition occurs when we subject ourselves to extended periods of sitting with little or no exercise. Venous blood then collects around the interconnecting network of veins surrounding our lower rectum and anal canal known as the "hemorrhoidal plexus." Blood that would normally flow back in veins through the pelvis, up through the liver, and forward along our abdominal wall swells out the sides of the hemorrhoidal plexus. Blood-filled sacs known as "hemorrhoids" balloon out into the anal canal, causing pain and bleeding. Long-distance truck drivers are one population especially prone to this condition. Sitting for long periods of time with no intervening periods of walking is a quite unnatural state for human beings. Hemorrhoid sufferers must begin to move. Unlike the legs, no artificial compression of the pelvis can assist blood return to the heart, although lying down and raising the level of the pelvis may help to some extent. Surgery again is a last resort, but individual prevention by exercising is the best therapy. It is simply what hominids have always done, and it is in the center of our adaptation as a species.

Mechanical Problems of the Arms and Shoulders

Our arms and shoulders are no longer involved in locomotion by suspending our body weight below tree limbs or supporting it on the ground via curled-up knuckles. Instead, our arms hang limply by our side when we walk, mimicking by their rhythmic swinging back and forth the quadrupedal gait of our distant ancestors. It is a rather impractical and even ridiculous mode of progression— waving limbs back and forth that do not even touch the ground— but there are significant evolutionary advantages. Our forelimbs became freed from moving our bodies around when we became bipeds, and were crafted by evolution to become exclusive manipulative organs. The anatomy of our arms and shoulders, however, is still that of an ape, and we can understand many of our shoulder ailments from this perspective.

The human hand has opposable fingers like those found in our primate relatives, the prosimians, the monkeys, and the apes. This five-digit hand structure is in itself remarkably primitive, recalling the condition in our far-off amphibian ancestors and still retained in modern frogs and salamanders. However, our hand muscles, neurological control of those muscles, and hand-eye coordination have evolved to a high degree of sophistication, belying our superficially "simple" hand structure. Primates in general and apes in particular use their hands to climb in the trees—a dangerous activity if you lose your hold—and to catch, pick, and convey to their mouths items of food (fruit, insects, berries, shoots of leaves, eggs, etc.). These two important biological functions of the primate hand are more than sufficient to explain the evolution of manual dexterity and the high degree of mobility that we have in our upper limbs.

Hominids added an additional function to the arm and the hand. They began to engage in a wide range of manipulative activities—tool use—that we know from the archaeological record has lasted for some 2.5 million years. Tool use as a major behavioral activity thus is even younger than bipedalism in our history as a species. We can develop orthopedic problems with our upper limbs if we stray too far from our apelike anatomical capabilities, such as by playing sports too long or too hard.

Our elbows and shoulders are joints that anatomically are made more for suspension than for industrial-strength power movements. In the "tool use" that constitutes hitting a tennis ball with force during a serve, our elbow joint acts as a pivot for a powerful extension of our arm. The ligaments and muscle tendons around our elbow joint are stressed in their abilities to hold the joint together and are commonly damaged. The fluid-filled bursas, cushioning the ligaments and tendons, become irritated and inflamed. We have a case of "tennis elbow."

Our shoulder has similar problems. Four small muscles surround our flat-surfaced shoulder-arm joint and rotate the arm around its long axis. In apes this wide range of movement allows the arm to adopt virtually any handhold. In humans it can get us in trouble if we exert too much force on these muscles. Baseball pitchers, for example, use these muscles—the so-called rotator cuff—to impart powerful spins to pitches delivered at speeds of over 90 miles an hour. Many pitchers experience pain and injuries to these shoulder muscles in the course of their professional pitching careers.

Between Scylla and Charybdis

A number of human orthopedic complaints can be traced back to a specific action, such as lifting a heavy box. But some common and preventable problems are due to work and leisure—too much activity and too little.

Not long ago, civilization was touted for bequeathing to modern people much more leisure time. But then cultural anthropologists studying living hunter-gatherers discovered that people like the San in southern Africa needed to engage in subsistence activities ("work") only a few hours a day. They had plenty of time to rest and pursue leisure activities.[6] Paradoxically, it is "civilized" people whose occupational activities have been integrated into the processes of industrial production, and whose patterns of occupational pathology reflect their specialized roles. Machinelike, repetitive work routines are especially prone to occupational injuries. Overuse of body parts in specialized ways, ones for which the human body was not designed by evolution, leads to structural failure, that is, very much the same as when machine parts wear out. This pattern of modern workplace injury has been termed "repetitive strain injury."[7]

Carpal tunnel syndrome is one such repetitive strain injury caused by too much work—work for which our bodies are not now suited. It is an inflammation of the muscle tendon sheaths that run under the strong fibrous band on the front of our wrists, the so-called flexor retinaculum. Like all the hominoids, we have strong arm and wrist flexor muscles. They evolved as part of our locomotor adaptation to tree life and were primarily designed to support our body weight when hanging or climbing on branches. Our wrist flexors thus evolved for "isotonic contraction" (muscle contraction against force that does not change the length of the muscle), rather than contracting to shorten the muscle. The flexor retinaculum is there to prevent "bowstringing" of our flexor muscles between the inside point of our elbow, where they attach to the bone, and their attachments to our finger bones. With repetitive flexing movements of our hand, as we might do in marathon typing or on an assembly line, our excessively moving flexor muscle tendons rub against the strong flexor retinaculum and become injured and inflamed. As the injured tendon sheaths swell, they put pressure on the nerve running with them under the flexor retinaculum through the wrist, the median nerve. Compression of the median nerve now causes muscle weakness and pain in the hand. At that point, we are forced to rest the hand and put on a volar splint to avoid movement of the wrist. As the swelling goes down, the pain and weakness subside—until we start back to work again.

On the other hand, so to speak, we have the lazy afternoon spent on the couch. In proper measure, rest and relaxation is perfectly healthy; but, all too often, chronic inactivity harms our musculoskeletal systems. When we do not move, the ligaments connecting the bones on the two sides of a joint contract, becoming tight and inflexible. The muscles that are supposed to move that joint also become shortened and weak. When the time comes that we finally do have to get up off the couch or out of bed, our lack of muscle strength and joint flexibility make moving a laborious task. In whatever job we do, our relatively small muscle mass is easily fatigued and overworked. The muscle fibers in certain muscle groups—for example, our shoulders—begin to spasm, and we have pain. This problem has become so common in America that a new disease has been invented for it—"fibromyalgia."

Fibromyalgia may or may not be a "disease" in the classical sense.[8] Its name derives from the connective tissue fibers that replace atrophied muscle tissue. But it is certainly real to the estimated 1.5 million Americans who suffer from it. The pain of fibromyalgia frequently is reported to be sited in "tender points" around the body. Neurological examination, however, consistently fails to locate nerve damage or underlying pathology. Fibromyalgia is frequently associated with stress and inflammation.

The genesis of fibromyalgia is inactivity. Muscles atrophy and joints become inflexible. When activity becomes unavoidable, a person moves, however unwillingly. Weak muscles and tight ligaments make fluid, coordinated movement difficult. With the increased weight that most inactive people are carrying, small muscle and ligament tears are common. In addition to the pain associated with the injury, these small-scale tears become inflamed and even more painful. Many tender points of fibromyalgia are likely caused by small-scale injury at major weight-bearing and lifting joints, such as the hip and the elbow. Other tender points are located at points of muscle tension, such as the shoulders. Without stretching and general mobility, these muscles become chronically contracted and painful.

Fibromyalgia is considered by many to be a mysterious disease, perhaps more psychosomatic or psychological in its origins than anything else. Others have hypothesized that it is an autoimmune disease—an attack of the body's own tissues by the immune system. And there is also the ever-present possibility that the disease is the result of invasion of the body by a pathogen, perhaps a virus. But the pattern of fibromyalgia is that of an "occupational disease"— one that is brought on by a person's particular pattern of work, behavior, and lifestyle. This interpretation is borne out by the finding that there is only one known therapy for fibromyalgia—activity. A planned regimen of stretching, movement, and strengthening exercises, along with lifestyle changes that reduce weight, allow better sleep patterns, and reduce stress, can totally eliminate the pain and stiffness associated with this ailment. In evolutionary terms, this treatment for fibromyalgia returns us toward the center of our adaptive landscape—somewhere out in the open, moving around, and not immobile in front of a television set.

Our modern lifestyle dilemma plays havoc with other systems of our body in addition to our musculoskeletal system. In the next chapter, we look at uniquely human (Level 16) diseases of civilization that affect our alimentary tract.

12

Gut Diseases

No one knows what to eat anymore. WeightWatchers tells you to cut out all the fat and most of the sugar in your diet, while the Atkins Diet says that you should eat meat and eliminate the carbohydrates.[1] The U.S. Department of Agriculture recommends six to 11 servings of bread and cereals per day[2] while the Origin Diet is based largely on cutting out all grain products from what you eat.[3] The U.S. Recommended Dietary Allowance (RDA) for vitamin C is 60 milligrams, but Nobel laureate Linus Pauling maintained that we should ingest 3,000 milligrams of vitamin C per day for optimum protection against disease and illness.[4] An evolutionary perspective gives us a scale on which to balance these very different recommendations.

Humans are a dietary paradox, embracing both sameness and variety. Sameness comes from the physiological imperatives of consistently fueling the body with reliable energy and nutrients, thus maintaining the homeostasis of the body. The main evolutionary advantage to early cells banding together to form multicelled organisms came from maintaining optimal feeding and living conditions of their ancestral sea environment. But much, much later, eating a wide variety of foods became the way that primates, and especially the hominids, maintained equilibrium in a changing environment on land. Climatic change placed our ancestors in situations where lush fruits, tasty insects, and tender food plants were in scarce supply. Those who survived adapted to eating a greater variety of foods—in habitats at which most nonhuman primates would have turned up their noses and then hightailed it back to the forest. We have evolved ways—anatomical, biochemical, physiological, and behavioral—to eat just about anything. We are true omnivores.

This very plasticity of food choice is now killing us because we have used it to specialize on marginal parts of our total potential diet. We have strayed too far from what we need to eat and have selectively chosen only a small part of the panoply of foods our ancestors ate.

Determining the adaptively normal human diet—our "ideal" nutrition—is only possible with an evolutionary approach. However, no other topic can touch such strongly held personal opinions and deeply seated emotions. We all feel quite resolute about what we want to eat and what is good for us. The lexical diversity of modern dietary lifestyle choices—vegetarian, vegan, organic, natural, lacto-ovo-vegan, low-fat, high-fiber, low-protein, Mediterranean—demonstrates the variety of possibilities. And each dietary strategy has its own rationale for providing the benefits of optimal health and long life. All cannot be right, and yet they cannot be all wrong. Millions of people seem to eat and live just fine, in the short term, with each of these diets. Many more millions are less fussy about their diet and just eat what the environment seems to provide—a Danish and coffee on the fly for breakfast, a fast-food burger for lunch, a quick takeout pizza for dinner. They begin to suffer the consequences in the short term.

Our goal in this chapter is to consider how our digestive system evolved and how it is adapted to function. We will then look at how modern diseases affect these adaptations and how we can prevent their ill effects.

Alimentary Anatomy

Our digestive tract begins with our mouth. Unlike many animals, humans do not use their lips, front teeth, and tongue for extracting food from the environment. We do not have the callused lips of the thorn-tree-eating black rhino, the piercing canines of the bloodsucking Mexican vampire bat, or the elongated sticky tongue of the anteater. Like all primates, we feed ourselves with our hands. As food goes into our mouth, it is dealt with by the teeth.

Teeth are of particular fascination to paleontologists, and tooth anatomy has played an important role in debates about classifying fossil species of animals. Virtually every cusp, wrinkle of enamel, groove, and millimeter of size difference in the known fossil teeth of hominids has been minutely examined. Stepping back from the detail, however, shows us that we humans, like most mammals, have four kinds of teeth: bladelike incisors in the front (two above and two below); puncturing canine teeth at the front corners of our mouth; three flat teeth in each row of teeth in the back of our mouth for crushing and grinding food (the molars); and two intermediate teeth, the premolars or bicuspids, between the canines and the molars.

Humans have small canines that do not project past the level of the other teeth, unlike our ape relatives. The apes use these teeth in feeding—usually to break open tough-skinned fruits or, in the case of gorillas, bamboo trees. They eat what is soft and delicious inside. The small size of human canines has been explained as an evolutionary by-product of tool use (with sharp tools replacing their puncturing function). Our canines now cut like incisors, scissorslike, against the canines in the opposite jaw. The resulting shearing battery of slicing teeth in the front of our mouth—incisors plus canines—is similar to the cutting "carnassial" premolars in carnivores. These meat-eating animals, like the dog, the cat, and the bear, which do not grasp their food in the hands, have retained their pointed incisors and puncturing canines. They have evolved scissorslike cutting in their cheek teeth. Prey is caught and killed with the front teeth and sliced up in the back teeth. In hominids, prey is delivered by the hands to the front teeth, already dead or at least incapacitated, and ready for eating. The front teeth slice the meat, and the back teeth process it. The anatomy of our front teeth shows an adaptation to meat eating in our ancestry.

Our molar teeth on the other hand are flat-topped, capped with thick enamel, impervious to cracking, and, most importantly, quite large. One of the main biological differences between humans and apes is that humans are "megadont"—more accurately, "megamylic"—meaning that they have big molar teeth in relation to their body size. Our molars are really the most important physical dietary adaptation that we have.

A human being watching the raw power of a feeding gorilla may feel that his or her chewing anatomy is far weaker. But this perception is not entirely correct. The gorilla has massive front teeth and huge temporal muscles covering the back of its skull, but humans have bigger and thicker-crowned molars that generate more force between them when we chew. Our temporal muscles are much smaller than those of the gorilla, but they are attached to the bone so that their mechanical pull is oriented directly above our molar teeth. We can crush objects between our molars that a gorilla has to swallow whole. Some extinct hominids, especially the robust australopithecines, had even bigger and thicker crowned molars than we do.

Some theorists have suggested that the hominid's strong chewing mechanism is an adaptation to herbivory—a diet of vegetation. John Robinson, a paleoanthropologist at the Transvaal Museum in South Africa and later the University of Wisconsin, pioneered in the 1960s the "dietary hypothesis" to explain the huge expansion in the size of the cheek teeth in robust australopithecines. He suggested that these hominids were vegetarians, emphasizing their chewing teeth like grazing and browsing African ungulates. Our ancestors, the gracile hominids leading to the Homo lineage, he considered omnivores. Proponents of a vegetarian natural diet for humans extended Robinson's ideas about the function of the molars from robust australopithecines to ourselves.

Later studies have shown that the function of our molar teeth is not limited to a specialized diet. They can pulverize almost anything, however tough—fibrous plants, uncooked meat—into tiny digestible fragments. And as anthropologist Charles Peters described it, there was a "competitive advantage of the megadonts" in the scramble for sustenance on the early African savanna.[5] In such dry, nonforested habitats, plants and their seeds tend to be covered with thick outer coverings to prevent them from drying out. Jaws and molars strong enough to chew up tough sources of protein, carbohydrate, nutrients, and calories spelled the difference between life and starvation.

Once a hominid's teeth have finished with chewing food, it is swallowed into the esophagus and enters the stomach. Our stomach is a simple bag of encircling muscles with an internal lining, one cell thick, known as the "mucosa." In addition to producing mucus, as its name implies, its cells also release hydrochloric acid and hormones, such as gastrin. The muscles in our stomach contract to squeeze and further break up the food, which then travels as a slurry into our small intestines, where bile and pancreatic enzymes are added to it for digestion. The small intestine absorbs nutritive elements, and the remaining indigestible components in what we ate moves on into the large intestine. We humans have a short colon (large intestine) with a small, blind pouch called the "cecum," from which water is absorbed from feces before they are excreted.

The significant anatomical aspect of our stomach and intestines is their simplicity. Our stomach is like that of a carnivore, built for quick processing of high-calorie, high-quality food, not requiring very much more processing before being passed on to the intestines for absorption. Humans have a relatively short length of small and large intestines—about 20 feet long. Herbivores have a much longer intestinal tract, and they have additional storage areas for further fermentation of tough-to-digest food. Our cecum is small, and our appendix is a vestige of its earlier size. Ungulates, on the other hand, have sacculated stomachs, divided into sections, and a large cecum, where food can stay until bacteria break down the indigestible cellulose. Cows even regurgitate part of their stomach contents and rechew it. Obligate vegetarian primates, such as the leaf-eating langur monkeys of Asia and colobus monkeys of Africa, and the leaf- and pith-eating gorillas, have ungulate-like digestive tracts. Food stays in their stomachs much longer, and fermentation by resident stomach bacteria breaks down the cellulose, which mammals do not have digestive enzymes for. One recent study of lowland gorillas in the Central African Republic showed that 57 percent of this species' energy derived from fermentation of fiber in its large intestine.[6]

Food passes through our intestines in about 24 hours, another similarity to carnivores. But if our more herbivorous primate relatives have slower "gut passage times" and longer intestines, and we ourselves have vestiges of a former, more vegetarian diet, when did the anatomical change to a more varied diet, with meat, occur?

The Expensive Tissue Hypothesis

The soft-part anatomy of ancient hominids unfortunately did not fossilize. So we do not have a direct measure of stomach size or intestinal length of australopithecines. Several clever studies, however, have convincingly shown that australopithecines had more guts than we do.

Leslie Aiello and Peter Wheeler were interested in whence the evolving human body took the resources to reallocate to the expanding and energy-hungry human brain. They proposed the "expensive tissue hypothesis" as an explanation.[7] They found that the evolving hominid body could ill afford to reduce its skeletal muscles, heart and circulatory system, skeletal system, kidneys, liver, and reproductive system. Only the digestive tract was a possible source for the energy, nutrients, and blood supply needed for the enlarging brain. But the body still needed the same amount of sustenance. The solution was higher-quality food that required less processing time and a shorter digestive tract. Animal protein in the form of vertebrate skeletal muscle, organs, insects, and eggs are nutrient- and calorie-rich food sources, and, ecologically speaking, they are high-quality foods. Hominids began making such foods a major part of their diet as soon as their teeth could handle the toughness of uncooked meat and insect cuticle.

Australopithecines had large, thick-enameled molars, the jaw structure and muscles to chew with force, a relatively enlarged brain with respect to that of their ape forebears, and, by informed inference, also a relatively reduced digestive tract and an increasing component of animal protein in their diet. Recently discovered australopithecine bone implements with microscopic wear from digging out termite mounds show that early hominids regularly dined on insects.

Other parts of australopithecine anatomy, however, show that they still had big bellies and longer intestinal tracts than modern humans. The rib cage of "Lucy," the 3.2-million-year-old partial *Australopithecus afarensis* skeleton, was carefully reconstructed by Peter Schmid of Switzerland and shown to be bell-shaped, like an ape. The australopithecine pelvis is known from numerous studies to have been wider and more open than in humans. Assuming that viscera filled the wide space between the diaphragm and the pelvis, we have a pretty clear indication that australopithecines had intermediate-length intestines, in line with their brain size, which was intermediate to humans and apes. They had diets with much higher fiber[8] content than a normal modern human diet, more like that of gorillas.

A 1.6-million-year-old *Homo erectus* skeleton from Narioko-tome, Kenya, shows a rib cage with the modern barrel shape. Pelvic form is also comparable to modern humans. Brain size in *Homo erectus* is four-fifths that of modern humans. From these various anatomical indications, we can deduce that hominids were omnivorous as early as 1.9 million years ago, when *Homo erectus* first appears in the fossil record. Cut marks on animal bones made by hominid stone tools date back to 2.5 million years ago and support this inference.[9]

The combination of big, tough molar teeth that pulverized any food into digestible bits and sharp cutting tools that could be fashioned and used to eat a wide range of foods constitutes a formidable adaptation. The acquisition of fire and cooking along the way only added to the wide range of potential food items on the human menu. Pleistocene hominids seemed to have eaten their way across the Old World and then into the New, probably hunting most large and slow, but meaty, species to extinction by the end of the Pleistocene.[10] The very power of this dietary adaptation carries with it danger.

Dangers of the Human Dietary Adaptation

Being able to chew up virtually any substance and swallow it makes us more susceptible to poisoning ourselves than other species. Most of what we eat is what we learned to eat as children and what is sanctioned by the actions of people around us—not necessarily what is best for us to eat from evolutionary and nutritional stand-points. Although we may become sick to our stomach and even vomit what is immediately poisonous, there is a danger that we will continue to eat foods that are marginal in quality and whose long-term cumulative effects may be negative. Lactose intolerance and celiac disease (sprue) are two diseases in this category. The various cancers of the digestive tract are closely related to the carcinogenic compounds that we ingest in our food and water. Substances in our food that adults may be able to tolerate can cause birth defects in our offspring (chapter 3).

We are also ever in danger of eating too much. If we can efficiently process virtually all foods, and the foods we particularly like are in abundant supply, what stops us from gorging? We do not seem to have a very effective built-in stop mechanism. What we do have is the sensation of fullness in our stomach and intestines after eating that communicates to the brain that we are no longer hungry. But if what we eat is so insubstantial in fiber that it is absorbed rapidly and our stomach is soon empty again, we will tend to resume eating when our body already has plenty of calories to run on. Obesity, discussed in chapter 9, and the diseases of bulimia and anorexia nervosa are directly related to this aspect of the current discordance between our dietary adaptation and our modern diet.

A third danger area of our unique dietary adaptation is emotional and physiological—involving the brain-gut connection, a unique communication between the largest set of nerve connections in our body—the brain—with the second largest concentration—in our stomach and intestines. Both nerve fibers and hormones connect our brain and our digestive system. This interaction is intimate at conscious and unconscious levels, and the complexity of the human brain makes it unique within the animal kingdom. We see a discordant interaction at work when, for example, our conscious brain chooses a red tomato, which passes the visual test for ripeness, at a standard North American supermarket, but then later we do not want to eat the tomato because we suspect from prior experience that it will not taste very good (our gustatory brain tells us, in fact, that it will taste like cardboard). Our conscious brain knows that we should eat the tomato to stay healthy and chalks up our lack of enthusiasm for eating the tomato to its having been picked before it had ripened on the vine. We realize that appearances have deceived us, but then our conscious brain overrides our unconscious, and we eat the tomato, anyway. In other cases, our emotions may be swayed toward eating unhealthy foods by reason of persuasive marketing or even their smells (such as those cinnamon roll shops in malls).

Another discordant arena between conscious and unconscious dietary adaptations involves emotional stress, an all-too-common commodity of life in industrialized societies. Emotions can override our digestive functions, playing an important role in digestive diseases from ulcers to irritable bowel syndrome. Evolution has produced a finely tuned balance between our brain and gastrointestinal system to coordinate conscious behavior and eating. We cannot allow it to be overridden by the stresses and emotional upsets of modern life if we are to remain healthy.

Reconstructing the evolution of human diet is more than an exercise in evolutionary biology and paleoanthropology. If we do not eat the way we evolved to eat, we get sick. A number of particularly irksome diseases of modern life are traceable to aberrations of diet, and they are preventable.

Air Bread, Intestines, and Teeth

Did you ever wonder why fiber in your diet is good for you, besides to keep you regular? The evolutionary transition from mushy-fruit-eating apes to savanna australopithecines that ate fibrous roots, seeds, and meat was a fundamental one. Not only did our teeth evolve to deal with the new hardness of our food, so did our gastrointestinal tracts. When our teeth became harder, our bowels became selective. They absorbed what nutrients were broken down sufficiently to pass through the intestinal wall and into the bloodstream, and then voided the rest. A lot of what early hominids ate was chaff—indigestible fiber that our intestines evolved to move out rather than let sit and ferment, like a gorilla. There were plenty of calories and nutrients in what was digested and absorbed to sustain the hominid on its daily rounds. The intestines became adapted to a certain bulk and consistency of food passing through. Although diet changed in *Homo erectus*, a significant amount of fiber is undoubtedly an intrinsic part of our dietary adaptation.[11]

"Refined" cuisine—light and airy dishes that "melt in your mouth"—have a high energy:satiety index.[12] To prepare these recipes—as in much of French cooking, for example—the coarse fiber in the ingredients has to be removed, and raw produce is traditionally well cooked and smothered in sauce (frequently dairy-based). Wheat used in these dishes is ground to flour by modern roller milling techniques so that it has no fibrous, external seed coat. In this perspective, any foods made with whole grains, such as Chinese or Indian rice dishes, Mexican maize- and bean-based cuisine, or Scottish oatmeal, is sniffed at as being "unrefined." Many Western societies began to give up their old-fashioned coarse foods in the late 19th century in favor of more processed foods. But undoubtedly, Americans have perfected the refining of foods—developing the ultimate in high-energy, high-fat, low-fiber, preserved, and containerized food that can be quickly eaten—bequeathing to world civilization "junk food."

What happens if you eat only foods with little or no fiber? First, if you are an adult, you either do not end up with enough in your stomach to feel satiated ("full") when you have eaten enough calories, or worse, you eat vastly more food and calories than you need just to fill up the space in your stomach. In either case, there are health consequences.

When you eat airy, processed food, it passes through your stomach quickly into the small intestines. Here the small particle size of what you ate is quickly absorbed, leaving only a small amount of indigestible fiber to pass on to the large intestines. The large intestines wait for the normal bulk to come into them from the small intestines, but it does not come. The smooth muscles in the walls of the large intestines contract in their effort to move the bolus of feces along, but there is too little bulk to act on. The relatively thin walls of the colon are placed under extreme pressure and begin to balloon out. These ballooned-out sacs of our colon are termed "diverticula," and colonoscopies show that one in four Americans have them. In about 20 percent of these people, the diverticula become inflamed and painful, and the condition is then termed "diverticulitis." If not corrected, inflamed diverticula can rupture and spread infection throughout the body cavity.

The same mechanism explains appendicitis. Fecal material is forced into the blind end of the cecum (by a process known by the alliterative name of "inspissation") and into the thin cavity of the appendix by the tremendous pressure of the large intestine. There it forms a "fecolith," which causes inflammation and infection; if not treated with antibiotics or surgery, it can also rupture into the body cavity, potentially causing death.

Diverticulitis and appendicitis are very rare or unknown in underdeveloped countries of the world, preferentially afflicting the more industrialized countries whose inhabitants eat Western-style diets. Most studies implicate a low-fiber diet with the diseases of diverticulitis and appendicitis.[13]

Our modern-day mushy food has one other significant negative effect on the front part of our digestive system—our teeth. Not only is our soft-part digestive anatomy adapted to tough, fibrous food, so are our teeth and gums. Hard chewing, enamel to enamel and enamel to food, caused a significant amount of microscopic wear on our ancestors' teeth. This wear took off a layer of bacteria on our tooth surfaces and prevented tooth decay. Not one of the several thousand australopithecine or early *Homo* teeth now known show any evidence of a cavity. Today, mouth bacteria tend to sit on our teeth, causing bad breath, gum disease, and tooth decay. We moderns have found that we can mimic the salutary dental hygiene effects of our ancient diet by artificially scouring our teeth with abrasive toothpaste and dental floss. There is, however, evidence from fossil teeth that hominids as early as *Homo habilis* used toothpicks.[14]

Irritable Bowel Syndrome

"Stomachache" is the most common gastrointestinal complaint that doctors hear. Abdominal pain is frequently associated with either constipation or diarrhea. These conditions are generally temporary and can be caused by eating new foods in new places; for example, when tourists get "travelers' diarrhea." Bacteria, usually just a different strain of our normal gut denizen, *Escherischia coli,* is the most common cause. But when abdominal pain, constipation, and diarrhea become chronic complaints, and no infectious, biochemical, or anatomical cause for the problem can be found, a frustrated doctor will diagnose "irritable bowel syndrome (IBS)." Both the patient and the doctor realize that the problem is real, but effective treatment has been elusive. Physicians, noting that stress is usually associated with irritable bowel syndrome, may consider the ailment a psychosomatic one and refer a patient for psychiatric counseling. But counseling has been found to be largely unsuccessful in relieving its symptoms.

More recent research shows that the pain in irritable bowel syndrome is caused by muscular spasm of the longitudinal bands of smooth muscle that ensheathe the large intestine. In normal digestion, involuntary contractions of this muscle squeeze out water for absorption by the large intestines and move feces along toward the rectum for voiding. In irritable bowel syndrome, there are not enough intestinal contents for the smooth muscle to work on, the colon contracts down to a very narrow diameter, and the muscles cramp. The intestinal contents move slowly down the colon, leading to either constipation (no bowel movements for days) or watery stools caused by the spasmodic contraction of the smooth muscle. Researchers found that when a balloon placed into the colon of a patient with irritable bowel syndrome was inflated, it was painful. The muscular wall of the large intestine is sensitive and sore from overcontracting and resists any stretch. The patient may even experience pain when the colon normally fills after eating.

The underlying cause of irritable bowel syndrome is similar to that for diverticulitis and appendicitis—a mismatch of colon anatomy and physiology with the bulk and fiber content of food. Emotional stress exacerbates the condition, even if it does not cause it, because it slows down digestion even more. Stress initiates the fight-or-flight physiological mechanisms of the body that prevent the colon from normally contracting. A dietary change that includes fibrous foods is the most effective treatment for the condition, but it must be done gradually to allow the large intestine to adjust.

Peptic Ulcer

Physicians, until recently, thought that "peptic ulcers"—open sores in the stomach lining and the first part of the small intestine, the duodenum—were the pathological results of too much stomach acid, in turn caused by too much emotional stress. In 1982, that all changed. Two Australian researchers discovered a new bacterium, *Helicobacter pylori*, that is frequently associated with gastric and duodenal ulcers. They were so enthusiastic about their new discovery that they infected themselves with it and showed that an inflamed stomach lining resulted. All the medical textbooks were rewritten, and peptic ulcer was moved from the category of "unknown etiology" to that of "infectious causation." One of the discoverers himself, B. J. Marshall, did caution that this move might be premature.[15] Nevertheless, antibiotics quickly became the primary medical treatment for peptic ulcer, replacing antacids and a bland diet. Antibiotics have proven effective for many sufferers, demonstrating that a bacterial cause is indeed part of the cause of the problem, but other considerations clearly show it is not the sole cause. Lifestyle factors are still an important part of the peptic ulcer picture.

Infection by *Helicobacter pylori* is widespread. In fact, most people in the world have this bacteria in their bodies. Upwards of 90 percent of Africans, for example, have been infected in infancy or childhood. Yet a negligible number of these infected people (only the ones in big cities who live a Western lifestyle) ever get an ulcer, indicating that lifestyle factors, particularly stress and increased production of gastric acid, are likely involved in causing the disease.

A further indication that bacterial infection is not the sole cause of peptic ulcers is that in industrialized countries, where infection by *Helicobacter* generally occurs later in life, the bacterium is more common in lower socioeconomic groups. The low-income population is the very one which gets the least number of ulcers. It is the more affluent, high-stress, "type A" personalities, who as a group have less *H. pylori* infection, who are most affected. In fact, a significant number of these people do not have any bacterial infection, and irritation of the stomach lining by aspirin and other similar medications may be part of the cause of peptic ulcers in these cases.

Inflammatory Bowel Disease

When there is tissue damage in our intestines, our body is adapted to respond to the most likely agent of damage during our evolutionary history, a parasite burrowing into the mucosal wall to gain entry into the bloodstream. White blood cells are dispatched via the blood to the site of damage and fan out into the tissue. Today they usually do not encounter a parasite. The intestinal damage has been caused by some other agent—by chronic muscular contractions or inflammation from an impacted diverticulum.

Millions of Americans are plagued by a condition known as inflammatory bowel disease (IBD). Sometimes the inside mucosal lining of the colon is eaten away by ulcers (so-called ulcerative colitis). Other times the lining of the digestive tract becomes damaged and then very thickened, a type of IBD known as Crohn's disease. Crohn's disease can affect the entire gut from mouth to anus, but it is most common in the last part of the small intestine, the ileum, just before it enters the large intestine at the cecum. Diarrhea, abdominal pain, and bleeding from the rectum are characteristic of both diseases.

There is no consensus on what exactly causes IBD. Some researchers think that these diseases are caused by an immune system turning on itself. But there is a lack of convincing association with other so-called autoimmune conditions, which would be expected. A long-term search for an infective organism to explain IBD has been fruitless. No convincing genetic or biochemical hypotheses of causation have been advanced.

The epidemiological pattern of IBD closely parallels those of irritable bowel syndrome, diverticulitis, and appendicitis. People who eat normal, non-Western diets do not get either ulcerative colitis or Crohn's disease. These are diseases of civilization, and they have a high environmental causative component to them. It is likely that the same dietary factors that cause the less severe (irritable bowel syndrome) or the more acute (diverticultis and appendicitis) problems also contribute to the chronic conditions of IBD.

Research on a small New World monkey, the cotton-top tamarin, has been important in understanding the underlying causes of ulcerative colitis. In the wild, about 13 percent of this species' population have a low grade of ulcerative colitis, probably more or less "normal" for the population and due to an inflammatory reaction to intestinal bacteria and parasites.[16] But when any of these monkeys are captured, moved to an enclosure, and fed a zoo diet (which with its refined, grain-based, and low-fiber constituency resembles a modern Western diet), 80 percent of them develop ulcerative colitis. What exactly causes ulcerative colitis in captive tamarins is still unclear, but, after ruling out infection, parasites, and other obvious possible causes, these studies show that diet and environment (including stress) are important in explaining the disease. Like humans who eat a refined diet and lead sedentary lives, captive tamarins develop ulcers in their colon. When there has been chronic inflammation from an ulcerated colon, a significant number of the tamarins go on to develop cancer. One-quarter of the captive monkeys underwent cancerous or precancerous changes in their intestines. Cancer is entirely unknown among these and other primates in the wild.

Cancer of the Gastrointestinal Tract

Colorectal cancer, seen first as elongated proliferations from the gut wall known as "polyps," is the second most common cause of death from cancer in the United States today, according to the Centers for Disease Control. Internationally, however, it shows the same pattern of absence outside the developed world as other "diseases of civilization." The U.S. National Cancer Institute warns that ulcerative colitis is associated with colorectal cancer, and as any chronic inflammation or irritation of cells in the body may be potentially carcinogenic, this connection between long-standing inflammatory bowel disease and eventual cancers of the digestive tract makes sense. This same disease association was predicted from the tamarin studies. In this chapter, we have traced back these end-stage diseases to associations with diverticulitis and irritable bowel syndrome, and all these conditions are in turn closely related to an evolutionarily abnormal diet, one low in fiber. Other dietary factors, such as excess fat and even meat, have been implicated, but the specific biochemical, genetic, and pathological steps leading to colorectal cancer have yet to be defined.[17] As expected, a number of gene mutations that free cancerous cells from their pact of cooperative cell functioning, such as *ras* oncogenes, are seen in colorectal cancer.

In addition to clear sites of irritation and inflammation within the gut on which we might focus as danger spots for cancer to develop, colorectal cancer occurs in people without a specific risk factor. Many are the suggestions that the increasing numbers of toxins in our world are causing increased cellular damage and thus higher probabilities of cancer. Our digestive systems are natural places to posit such effects. If our feet and hands are our primary physical contact points with the environment, our digestive tract is our largest body surface in direct physical contact with the environment, especially from microbiological and biochemical points of view.[18] We ingest a veritable zoofull of organisms with every swallow, and the chemicals and trace elements that we eat so closely match our surroundings that we might as well have directly licked what we touch with our hands and feet. Our immune systems are adapted to deal with most organisms that we ingest, but man-made toxins are an evolutionary novelty. Epidemiological studies that might prove associations between specific toxins and colorectal cancer have so far been inconclusive.[19] But considering the cumulative effect of the many toxins in our modern environment and our lack of evolved mechanisms to deal with such foreign substances, it is not surprising that long-term cellular irritation and damage might result in cancer. The modern low-fiber diet, with its increased gut passage time, exacerbates any such toxic effects in our intestines because colon contents reside there a much longer time. A high-fiber diet is a good preventive strategy against colorectal cancer as well as the digestive diseases that are contributory to its development.

13

The Evolution of Psychiatric Disorders

Charles Darwin's third and last great, general work, after the *Origin of Species* and *Descent of Man*, was *The Expression of the Emotions in Man and Animals*.[1] The publication of this volume in 1872 marks the beginnings of the science of ethology, the study of the biology of behavior, and its later offshoot, sociobiology. Darwin recognized that in addition to anatomical structures, behavior—how those structures are used in everyday life—also had to evolve. He attempted to answer such questions as why chimps do not cry and why certain breeds of pigeons do barrel rolls when they fly.

Ethologists have attempted to render Darwin's insights scientifically measurable and testable, but the search for rigor in behavioral research has been difficult. Ethologists measure the time a behavior takes to perform in a natural setting (laboratory experiments are generally eschewed in ethology in preference to naturalistic field observation). They also observe what muscles are used in the behavior and what measurable differences there are in the results of the behavior—for example, the differences in the calls of songbirds. The discovery of units of inherited behavior, called "fixed action patterns," such as the clinging behavior of newborns discussed in Chapter 3, has been important in demonstrating that as Darwin hypothesized, behavior is genetically inherited. Ethologists and sociobiologists use the comparative approach in studying the evolution of behavior.

Human behavior has also been studied extensively and in depth by sciences other than biology, specifically cultural anthropology (ethnology), psychology, and other social sciences. These fields have focused not on the simple, animal-like behaviors of human beings, but rather on their most complex and highly evolved behaviors—religion, taboos, kinship, law, economics, and language. Like the proverbial six blind Indian wisemen observing an elephant, each one promotes its limited view of humanity as basic, essential, and supportable by its set of observed facts. The social sciences have emphasized the learned component of human behavior—the part that is not inherited and is acquired by people as members of social groups. The aggregate of this learned behavior that is passed on from one generation to the next is termed "culture," a concept developed by cultural anthropology. In truth, all observations about human behavior have to be compatible with an integrated understanding of the human organism, an organism that did indeed evolve out of simpler life-forms.[2] This chapter will look at human behavior as an evolved and integrated complex between biology and culture. When aspects of the adaptation fail, behavioral dysfunction— mental illness—results.

Interestingly, the new field of evolutionary medicine has had its greatest impact in psychiatry, the medical field dedicated to studying and treating mental illness. Perhaps this is because psychiatrists and psychologists have begun to abandon the long-held theoretical underpinnings of Freudian and behavioral psychology, which they have been found to be too limited for adequately dealing with the range of modern psychiatric disorders. An evolutionary approach does indeed seem to provide extremely promising new preventive measures and therapies for treating mental illness.

Establishing the Baseline:
Modern Humankind as a Captive Animal

Darwin first noted that people were self-domesticated—with ear muscles once needed for picking up auditory danger signals (just like sheep and floppy-eared domestic dogs) now degenerate, a decreased sense of smell, and eyesight tending towards myopia. Zoologist Desmond Morris, in his 1969 book *The Human Zoo*, took Darwin's thesis further and applied it to human behavior.[3] Morris compared humans to captive baboons, the males of which kill each other when crowded together, and zoo animals, which show repetitive, rhythmic behavior, masturbate, and usually fail to parent their offspring, even if they succeed in reproducing. The same species show none of these behaviors in the wild.

Two aspects of the behavior of animal species in the wild, in particular, are violated by zoo environments: territory and hierarchy. These evolved mechanisms keep animal species organized in the wild. Highly territorial animals will defend every bit of the ground, tree, or water space that they occupy, while less territorial species will tolerate incursions. Either way, the behavior serves to spread out individuals and groups within the species so that there is a more or less even distribution over the habitable range of the species.

Hierarchies are ordered behavioral arrays of individuals within a group. For example, when you stand in line at the grocery store, you are tacitly agreeing to allow the person in front of you to go first through the checkout counter. Hierarchies used to be considered primarily relevant to dominance interactions, and they were colloquially termed "pecking orders" because they had first been observed in birds. Hierarchies actually have the effect of reducing aggression in a group because they use a preset ordered arrangement to determine access to resources, such as food, water, sex, sitting places, and grooming by other members of the group. Aggressive interactions happen only when there are challenges to the hierarchy. Dominant individuals have a shutoff valve for aggression when lower-ranking individuals show submissive behavior. A cowering dog, for example, will not be attacked by the leader of the pack.

What happens in a primate group with extreme crowding and disruption of normal territoriality and hierarchy was shown vividly by a study of captive baboons in the 1930s by British anthropologist Solly Zuckerman.[4] A large group of baboons captured in East Africa was put into cages and sent by ship to England for study. A number of the males were killed by other males during the trip. When the baboons arrived, Zuckerman studied their behavior and was struck by the aggressive interactions between the male baboons. Trying to deduce what they were competing for, he concluded that it was sex. The males who won the battles mated with the females, usually several, in the group. It was easy to translate baboon behavior into a metaphor for human male competition for female attentions, with due consideration given to the societal conventions and trappings of civilization that must have intervened since the evolutionary divergence of baboon and man.

Primatologists and social scientists now generally recognize that Zuckerman's observations on the captive baboons, while accurate, were not representative of normal baboon behavior. Ethological studies of wild baboons in Africa pioneered by anthropologist Sherwood Washburn in the 1960s showed a much more sedate and well-ordered group—not the manic, sex-crazed killer monkeys that Zuckerman recorded. Hierarchy and territoriality were important organizing themes among the baboons, keeping the peace and making normal life possible. Only when they became disrupted did all hell break loose.

There are lessons here for human beings, but they have not often been heeded. Psychologist Frederick Goodwin, for example, was head of the U.S. Alcohol, Drug Abuse, and Mental Health Administration when, in 1992, he gave a lecture attempting to shed light on the pattern of aggression, antisocial behavior, and exaggerated territoriality of urban street gangs. He attempted to draw a parallel between primatological studies such as Zuckerman's and the crowded conditions of our inner cities, but unfortunately he did not choose his words well. The Congressional Black Caucus immediately called for Dr. Goodwin's resignation because his remarks had been interpreted as an unflattering comparison between predominantly black urban youths and African baboons. Although explanations were given, Goodwin was reassigned to another agency, and the point he was trying to make was forgotten.

What Dr. Goodwin failed to convey was that *any* human being, *all* of us of ancient African heritage, when stuck captive in the sweltering heat of a concrete-and-asphalt urban zoo in summer, would similarly turn on the fire hydrants in the streets to cool off. The extreme hierarchical loyalty and the violent defense of territory seen in urban gangs are exactly the behavior we would expect of a social primate like ourselves placed in a marginal environment. Less violent—but no less vicious—arenas are the corporate office and the government bureaucracies, with workers corralled into cubicles and stifled in mundane jobs while vying for favor from above, greater supervisory capabilities, and bigger offices— that is, for better mates, dominance, and territory. Perhaps we should regard more highly the lives of wild-living, savanna-adapted, African higher primates. After all, it is also our basic adaptation. Although baboons come by this ecological specialization separately from hominids, because they evolved from forest-living monkey ancestors, we share with our baboon cousins an appreciation of open vistas, fresh air, the smell of the coming rain, the shade of trees, and the wonderful wetness of a cool water hole on a hot afternoon.

Congested cityscapes are only the most egregious of the abnormal urban environments that modern people have fashioned for themselves. Like the evolutionarily abnormal biological conditions that we have seen predispose us to physical disease, abnormal social and environmental conditions lead to psychological ills.

Depression and Suicide

Depression is so common in modern-day America that it has been described as an epidemic. The ghosts of our hardworking grandparents must be shaking their heads in disbelief that despite all that we seem to have, we are so depressed. But it is not what we have accumulated materially, but rather what we have lost, that leads to depression.

Americans truly do not understand depression. They prefer to act, solving problems by doing. Given an option, most Americans would like to keep busy working on the wrong solution, then do it right only after being forced by trial and error, even if analysis beforehand (or reading the instructions) would have saved much time, money, and effort. Depression, by making such an activist approach impossible, is anathema to the American spirit. Lack of activity when nothing physically is wrong with you is more likely to elicit hostile, silent tolerance than emotional support from your family and friends, not to mention coworkers. Treatments have ranged from extensive psychotherapy to frontal lobotomies. Today, electroshock and drugs help to control depression, but it can destroy lives. What is it, and how do we understand it?

Humans are adapted to living in small social groups, between around 25 to 100 people, most of whom they know from birth until death, and many of whom they are related to. Much of everyday human social behavior is based on predictions of other people's reactions. These predictions are apt to be very accurate when they are rooted in a lifetime of experience. We know who owes us a favor, who will be particularly hard-nosed about an obligation, who will cut us some slack, who we can visit with for a good laugh, and who we can count on in a crunch. We know who peoples' parents and grandparents are, where they live, what happened in their lives to make them the way they are, and why we like or dislike them.

But what happens when we live in a virtually anonymous society where we know no one? We lack a rich background knowledge in our social interactions, calling many of our assumptions about society into question and making our presumed social contracts uncertain—which accounts in part for our increasingly litigious society. We also lack the high-quality emotional feedback that such in-depth social interactions bring us. Most of us, however, connect ourselves with a group of a hundred or so individuals with whom we normally interact—our surrogate ancient hominid tribe. These friends and relatives may be far-flung, but we stay in contact via telephone, e-mail, an annual holiday letter, and the odd trip through town. Nondepressed hominids these days seem to be able to deal with most issues of time and space in regard to their dispersed tribal contacts without too much difficulty, but for most, having their mate and/or nuclear family close at hand is still critical for mental health and happiness.

Issues of hierarchy today are somewhat different. It is undoubtedly much healthier to be a big fish in a small pond. In the ancient hominid world, everyone was a fish of some size—sometimes a big fish, sometimes a medium-sized fish, or sometimes a little fish—but the pond was always small. Everyone was noticed as some type of fish. Everyone had a place and an identity. Like baboon society, the hominid social hierarchy established order and harmony in the daily workings of the tribe. But in the modern world, the pond is potentially ocean-sized, and one fish can easily become lost in its vastness. When individuals do not feel that they have a place, a role, or an identity that matters to anybody—that is, they do not exist within a social hierarchy—they become listless, they lose interest in most of the activities of life, and they stop interacting with other people. In short, they become depressed. When humans' evolved social adaptations fail, submitting to chronic depression is as understandable a response, but just as unacceptable, as engaging in gang violence.

Depression is an evolved biopsychological adaptation within a social primate group setting. It is associated with various changes in brain chemistry. Levels of serotonin in the brains of monkeys drop as their hierarchical status in the group becomes lower. Serotonin is an ancient neurochemical, perhaps a billion years old,[5] that inhibits the transmission of nerve impulses across synapses in the brain. It counteracts the excitatory actions of adrenalin and dopamine. Calm, dominant monkeys have high levels of serotonin, while high-adrenalin, lower-ranking monkeys tend to be more excitable, aggressive, stressed, and prone to depression. Captive or crowded conditions essentially create a population of only low-ranking individuals, with concomitant higher levels of depression. We can also see why, when the evolved interaction of the serotonergic and dopaminergic systems is out of balance, hyperactivity and mania are frequently associated with depression.

In depression, human behavior becomes submissive, like a cowering dog. Body posture and facial expression both convey a social message of pitifulness. Slumped shoulders, a down-turned mouth, and contraction of the corrugator muscles at the inner edge of the eyebrows (forming a characteristic triangular skin wrinkle known as Veraguth's fold) are panhuman indicators of depression. They are silent supplications for consolation, help, and camaraderie from the social group. After a loss of status or some other blow to their self-confidence, such as a major injury, illness, or loss of a close relative, individuals may benefit from a depressive episode. The social signals of depression elicit empathetic social interaction, eventually reintegrating depressed primates into the group, with new friendships and alliances.

The social functions of depression may be lost, however, if there is no one there to notice. In modern society, where your ancient hominid tribe may be dispersed over thousands of miles and connected to you only episodically and mainly by electronic means, it is possible for you to sustain a major emotional blow and have no one around to notice or care about the folds over your eyes. With the fast pace of modern life, changes in hierarchy are common, families are small, deaths of family and close friends hit hard, and depression is rampant.

There can also be a physical aspect of the adaptiveness of depression. Depression frequently follows significant stress and trauma. For example, postpartum depression may follow the physical ordeal of birth. Posttraumatic stress syndrome is a depressive state that may follow wartime physical trauma, the amputation of a limb, or any extremely difficult emotionally traumatic experience. Depression in these circumstances is physiologically adaptive, allowing the individual to withdraw from the normal social milieu and recuperate.

The evolved and adaptive nature of depression is also shown in cases in which a depressed state actually precedes potentially stressful situations. Such an anticipatory depression occurs in seasonal affective disorder (SAD), a state of long-term depression that sets in during the dark, cold days of winter, only to dissipate when days become longer and warmer in spring. SAD affects mostly women, who make up between 60 percent and 90 percent of the patients diagnosed with this disorder. It is exclusively a condition seen in high latitudes with marked seasonal variation. SAD is reasonably interpreted as an adaptation that acts to keep individuals close to home, expending little energy, and probably not conceiving children (it, like other depressive disorders, extinguishes interest in sex) during the harsh winter months. Only in spring does a young man's (and a young woman's) fancy brightly turn to thoughts of love. This adaptation, although not the romanticist's vision of Stone Age lovemaking on cave-bear skins spread before a roaring fire in wintertime, was undoubtedly advantageous in the normally prevailing seasonal environments in the nontropical parts of the world populated by hominids over the past 2 million years.

Even if depression is an evolved adaptation, it is not fun when you have it. Can it be prevented? Should it be prevented?

The answer to the first question is a qualified yes. If a patient has recurrent or chronic depression, a psychiatrist can prescribe a drug, a serotonin-specific reuptake inhibitor (SSRI), that elevates serotonin in the synapses of the brain. Like high-ranking monkeys, the individual so treated loses the postures and expressions of depression, becomes active, and resumes social roles. Use of SSRIs to relieve the transient effects of depression is defensible, but these drugs do not take away the underlying causes of chronic depression and should not be prescribed for long-term maintenance. To cure depression, we must reestablish the lost nexus of our hominid social past. As clear as that goal may be, it will be a challenge for modern evolutionary psychiatry, as well as modern society as a whole, to achieve. Some radical solutions are proposed in the next chapter.

Evolutionary Psychology of the Triune Brain

The evolution of the brain must be important in understanding its dysfunction, but neither fossil studies nor molecular researches have so far provided much guidance. Comparative neuroscience studies have been the most helpful. Neuroscientist Paul MacLean of the National Institutes of Health studied the brain function and behavior of reptiles, monkeys, and humans in his development of the evolutionary theory of the triune brain.[6] "Triune" means "three in one," and MacLean used the term to mean that the human brain exists as a single functioning entity, even though it has sublevels that continue to function as ancestral brains. He called these the reptilian brain (our Level 9), the paleomammalian brain (Level 10) and the neomammalian brain (Levels 11 through 17). The triune brain model explains not only a lot of why our brains function the way they do, but why our treatments of mental illness work as well as they do.

The reptilian brain, called by MacLean the "R-complex," is to be found in the modern human brain buried beneath the huge expansion of gray matter known as the "cerebral hemispheres." Anatomically, it consists of the ancient, unpaired brain structures of the brain stem—the cerebellum, the medulla oblongata, the pons, and the midbrain (including the substantia nigra), as well as the most primitive of the paired structures of our brains—the olfactory bulbs (the "smell brain," the most primitive part of our cerebrum), and the oldest basal nuclei, the globus pallidus. Our reptilian brain is alive and well in us; its basic functions, however, have just been refined by evolution. For example, when a man detects the perfume of a woman who steps into an elevator with him, his reptilian brain may direct him to attempt to mate with her, but his paleomammalian brain moderates his behavior by interpreting the smell as positive, assessing the situation emotionally, recognizing the woman as unfamiliar, and deeming overt mating behavior as inappropriate under the circumstances. The neomammalian brain may then direct the man to smile in an appropriately cordial manner, or even to say, "Nice fragrance." The reptilian brain, by extension from observations of the behavior of reptiles, directs the components of our behaviors that are patterned, ritualistic, and rigid. They are the parts of the brain that maintain hierarchy and territoriality. When they malfunction, they can account for symptoms of paranoia, depression, and obsessive-compulsive disorders. Parkinson's disease, a neurological tremor caused by inadequate dopamine in cells of the substantia nigra, is sited within the R-complex.

The paleomammalian brain consists of what MacLean termed in 1952 the "limbic system"—all paired structures within our cerebrum that include the hypothalamus,[7] the hippocampus,[8] and the amygdala.[9] "Limbic" refers to the "margins" around the brain stem and was first used by the great French anthropologist and anatomist Paul Broca to refer to a limbic lobe of the brain. The limbic system "interprets" many of the directives of the R-complex—mediating emotions and feelings such as fear, rage, pain, love, and sexual attractiveness. The R-complex may direct that it is time to eat, but the limbic system decides what would taste good. Alzheimer's disease affects the limbic system, causing a decrease in cells and neurofibrillary tangles in the amygdala, which cause a number of emotional disturbances, and a loss of cells in the hippocampus, which causes memory loss.

The neomammalian brain, sometimes called just the "neo-cortex," is the only part of the brain that is endowed with language—but only one-half of it. The neocortex is also unique in that it is lateralized; that is, the left and right hemispheres have different functions. The left hemisphere controls the right half of the body, receives sensory information from the right side of the body, and usually has the speech centers. The right hemisphere is similarly connected to the left side of the body and is usually mute, being more adept at solving complex three-dimensional problems and maintaining a global awareness. Logical functions, mathematical ability, verbalization, writing, art, and music are all functions of the neocortex. Strokes—blockages of small blood vessels that cut off blood flow to a part of the brain—mainly affect the neocortex and are seen as muscle paralysis or difficulty in speech production.

The model of the triune brain is a useful and important way of understanding evolutionary psychology, even if further research extends the number of its levels or shows that there are many and intimate connections among the levels. There are, for example, certainly lower reaches of the brain than the R-complex, and we can expect future research to uncover these fish and invertebrate brains. And many of the primordial functions of the levels of the brain may be expected to have been altered by evolution for current functions. This is why, when a higher-level brain function is knocked out, we do not function exactly as a nonprimate mammal or a reptile might behave.

When speech centers of the neocortex (Broca's and Brodmann's areas) suffer nerve cell death from a blocked artery during a stroke, our abilities to talk or understand words are impaired. But the remainder of our brains continue to function, and we can still think and feel. Neocortex functions are deficient in Down's syndrome patients and other "mentally retarded" individuals. Depression and mania may be primarily paleomammalian (limbic system) disorders. This is where serotonin in the brain is produced, and this is the emotional center for many of the symptoms of depression and paranoia. Obsesssive-compulsive disorders may be sited primarily in the R-complex, but with ramifying connections to higher brain levels. Serotonin is a neurotransmitter that links the R-complex in the brain to another major body system, the gastrointestinal tract.

Eating Disorders

Recent discoveries about the body's production of serotonin have been surprising. Serotonin is mostly produced not in the paleo-mammalian cortex of the brain, but in the gastrointestinal tract by a parallel "brain"—the enteric nervous system.[10] This "gut brain" has some 100 million neurons and is as large as the spinal cord, producing all the same neurotransmitter chemicals as the central nervous system. It produces serotonin when the gut is full, com-municating to the brain a sense of well-being. As we have seen, high serotonin levels in the body correlate to a high position in the group hierarchy. How did such an unusual system evolve, and what happens when it goes awry?

For our entire evolutionary history, availability of food has been a determining factor in our reproductive success, in turn the most important aspect of our fitness in evolutionary terms. If we are not well fed, it makes very good adaptive sense to feel "down" so that we do not challenge the dominant individual in the group on that day. If we are well nourished and full of energy, on the other hand, serotonin levels assist us in our soaring ambitions, and we feel like we can conquer the world.

The gut-brain axis explains why eating disorders are associated with anxiety and depression. Social pressures in the Western indus-trialized societies can lead individuals to eat little or nothing in order to grow ever thinner. This mental disorder, anorexia nervosa, is particularly common in adolescent females. One of its first man-ifestations early in this century was seen in nuns who attempted to subsist only on the wafers of unleavened bread and a single swallow of wine that they received at Communion. In anorexics, the neo-cortex overrides the lower levels of the triune brain to deny the body food. But the lower levels revolt, causing severe depression.

A related disorder is bulimia—"binge-eating" followed by induced vomiting. The population at risk is the same—adolescent females. Body weight in bulimics, however, may be normal, whereas anorexics are emaciated. Both groups think of themselves as overweight, taking to heart the saying that you can "never be too thin." They suffer from malnutrition, vitamin deficiencies, bleeding gums, poor complexions, and gastrointestinal difficulties, particularly constipation.

Anorexia and bulimia are considered here illnesses of Level 17, modern human society, because their underlying cause is a societally induced, dysfunctional body-image ideal. It is also possible to think of them as a by-product of a toxic diet—poisoned with so much sugar and low-fiber carbohydrate that even eating enough calories to fulfill your daily needs leaves you still hungry and your stomach virtually empty. Anorexics and bulimics have just decided that if they are going to be hungry anyway, why not at least be thin and socially acceptable? This is obviously not the answer. Rather, a low-calorie diet that tastes good, in keeping with evolved adaptations, is possible. Such a diet is discussed in the next chapter. Food must meet our nutritional and metabolic needs, keeping our R-complex going. It should fill us up, keeping our gut brain happy. It should taste good, thus keeping our paleomammalian brain satisfied. And finally, it should serve our longer-term, societal goals, thought out by our neocortex.

Attention Deficit Hyperactivity Disorder

We have seen that mania is a partner with depression in low-status, crowded, and stressful primate group settings. Manic behavior can also have another cause—a physiological response to an abnormal environment. Too many tasks to perform, too much stimuli to respond to, or inadequate time to complete behaviors all cause stress. A common response to stress of this nature is hyperactive, poorly directed, and incoherently thought-out speech and behavior.

Perhaps the most abnormal environmental condition to which we are subjecting ourselves and our children is nervous system overload. Like most mammals, the human senses are adapted to exquisitely sensitive perception of environmental stimuli, which are important environmental cues for such activities as avoiding predators and catching animal prey. Inundating a mammal with excessive environmental stimuli and asking the brain and neuronal circuits to do too much produces neurosis, a conclusion that the great Russian psychologist Ivan Pavlov discovered in 1928. Dogs required to discriminate differences between more and more similar objects eventually became hyperactive, extremely agitated, and unmanageable whenever presented with the experiment. The neurosis is learned and entirely environmental in causation. Pavlov termed it "experimental neurosis," but he unwittingly put his finger on a major cause of modern mental illness.

Modern human life is a cacophony of sounds, lights, movements, and exhortations to do something—buy something, go somewhere, quit what you are doing and do something else. For adults, who grew up with some version of all this racket and have gotten used to it, a lot is tuned out—either ignored consciously or edited out at the level of the thalamus in the brain, very much like the hum of an air conditioner. Some of us use the mute button on our remote control a lot. But the environmental assaults have gotten much worse, and for newly minted people with unhabituated nervous systems—children—the noise can be overwhelming. Take a look at just the speed with which the images are flashed on the screen in many children's television shows. Adults around them talk so fast they cannot be understood. Many children almost never walk anywhere—they are whisked to their next appointment at freeway speeds, again with everything whizzing past. When modern children "relax," they play electronic games whose object is to push buttons frenetically in response to rapidly moving objects on a screen. Because the games become progressively more difficult as the child plays, he or she not infrequently ends by slamming the game down or banging the keyboard in frustration. Pavlov would recognize the behavior.

Attention deficit hyperactivity disorder (ADHD) is now the most commonly diagnosed mental disorder in American children.[11] Its proliferation is so recent that many general psychiatry and medical textbooks do not even index the term. Its symptoms are an inability to sit still or to pay attention for more than a few seconds at a time, constant and uncontrollable hyperactivity, and, for lack of a better term, obliviousness. Kids with ADHD just seem to be off in their own world, unreachable. ADHD has become the bane of the public schools because affected children are so disruptive. The condition is treated with a mild neurological stimulant drug called Ritalin, now by far the most widely prescribed children's drug in America. Many thousands of children are drugged before they can go to school in the morning and must be maintained in that state to be manageable. Ritalin sounds a lot like soma, the hypothetical drug conjured up by Aldous Huxley in his 1932 novel *Brave New World* to keep society under control, except that Ritalin is just used on children.

Although psychiatrists and psychologists have been unable to agree on the causes of ADHD,[12] an evolutionary perspective makes a presumptive explanation possible. ADHD seems to be a rather normal response for a juvenile primate placed in a very abnormal environment. Primates learn by playing, usually rough-and-tumble play. Primates are also highly social animals. Inactive, isolated lifestyles typify the ADHD child and set the stage for the syndrome to develop. Humans are the brainiest of the primates, and to offset the lack of play or social stimulation, ADHD children turn to undirected self-play and fast-paced, short-attention-span sources of stimulation. Neurosis sets in with the flood of stimuli that overload neural circuits. ADHD is classified as a Level 14 disorder because it is a basic failure of the higher primate level of social organization.

Unfortunately, children do not just grow out of ADHD. The hyperactivity abates with age, but the lack of ability to focus the mind and stay on task remain. ADHD in adults will become an increasingly common ailment as the percentages of the school age population with the disorder continue to climb. Adult ADHD represents a major impediment to career advancement in an age of an increasingly highly trained workforce. With a daily dose of Ritalin, an ADHD adult can usually function at some level, but far below his or her potential optimum. A much better solution is to prevent ADHD in the first place, and that requires evolutionarily aware lifestyle changes early in a child's development.

Inherited Phobias and Schizophrenia

Depression and ADHD seem to be adaptive responses of our brain to abnormal environmental conditions. They are diseases of civilization, virtually unknown in other cultures and in earlier times. Although genetic components play roles in depression and ADHD, these mental illnesses are in large part acquired.

Another class of mental illness is different. These are phobias or psychiatric conditions that people are born with. Specific genes that are responsible for them have so far eluded science, but they seem to exist worldwide at about the same rate of occurrence. Either almost everyone has them to some extent, like a fear of heights, or a constant percentage of a human population is born with the condition, as in schizophrenia, which occurs in about 1 percent of all populations worldwide. There are two evolutionary explanations for inborn psychiatric disorders. They are (or were) adaptive to life, or they are an evolutionary cost incident to other benefits that their genes confer.

Phobias are inborn fears that natural selection has conferred on the survivors of countless encounters with death over the millennia. A lazy lemuroid lounging in the late afternoon sun who did not react to a nearby boa constrictor ended up as dinner, and did not pass on any more of its genes to subsequent generations. A juvenile hominoid who was just too fearless went out on a slippery limb, fell, and died of a broken neck. He also did not pass on his genes to any progeny. The relatives of these individuals, a little more fearful of snakes and heights, survived and passed on their behavioral characteristics, which included a healthy respect for things ancestrally dangerous.

Unusual phobias are a standard of talk shows. Some people, it seems, are afraid of anything. For example, triskaidekaphobia is fear of the number 13, arachnophobia is fear of spiders, and atychiphobia is fear of failure. You will not find most of these phobias in a psychiatry textbook, not only because they are highly idiosyncratic and mostly learned, but, more importantly from a medical standpoint, they do not seriously impair normal daily functioning. But a number of fears are consistent enough to suggest that they are hard-wired into our brains. Fear of loud noises (ligyrophobia), heights (acrophobia), the sight of blood (hematophobia), the dark (nyctophobia), and reptiles (herpetophobia) are all understandable from a standpoint of our ancestral heritage from our tree-living forebears. They really cause us psychiatric problems only when they become magnified and exaggerated. Normally, we can avoid all the stimuli that may set them off, and these fears are adaptive.

Schizophrenia is different. The term literally means "split mind," but it is not the mental illness commonly known as "split personality." Rather, there is a dissociation of an individual's mind with reality. Schizophrenics may hear voices in their heads, feel that they are being pursued, or stare into space, motionless. Their mental state disrupts their social and family relationships and represents a major impairment to their daily functioning. Schizophrenics may be very creative and imaginative in the alternate world that they create in their minds. This creativity may be the key to understanding the evolutionary origins of the disease.

Human evolution is typified by an extremely rapid increase in the size of the brain, but paleoanthropologists have always been hazy about what exactly has evolved. Is it "extra neurons," as Harry Jerison thought,[13] or increased connections between association areas, or increased storage area for memory, or more processing gray matter for language and toolmaking? Schizophrenia may actually be a good clue as to what actually evolved in the human mind over the last several millions of years—just in exaggerated form. Perhaps it was creativity—the ability to make up an alternative way of looking at things, regardless of the subject. T. J. Crow has suggested that schizophrenia is a by-product of the evolution of language and its localization within the left cerebral hemisphere.[14] Another hypothesis explains the persistence of schizophrenia genes in the human population by a supposed selective advantage enjoyed by "Odyssean personalities"—those with schizoid-paranoid personalities.[15] L. F. Jarvik and B. S. Deckard suggest that "in a world plagued by terror, strife, and war, they, rather than their trusting peers, are the ones more likely to survive long enough to ensure the survival of their progeny." Whatever the exact selective advantages of schizophrenia genes, the potential evolutionary advantages of an adaptation conferring new ways of thinking to a population of hominids facing a rapidly changing set of Plio-Pleistocene environmental conditions is tremendous. Schizophrenia may be just the 1 percent genetic load that goes along with the overall adaptive advantage of the large and complex human brain.[16]

This view of schizophrenia fits with the way most cultures around the world treat schizophrenics. They tolerate them. They ascribe to them the status of seers, shamans, and magicians, and they use their altered views of reality to assess their society's adaptations. In today's complex Western world, the status of schizophrenics has been taken over by research scientists, whose thought processes are similarly not understood by the general public but whose pronouncements are listened to. Actual schizophrenics are isolated and ignored, their messages from the other side of the rational divide no longer listened to. Suicide rates are high in schizophrenics, between 15 percent and 20 percent, and the only treatment is pharmacological maintenance in a state of mental suspended animation. Schizophrenics are rarely dangerous to society, and better solutions need be found for their treatment.

The Phenomenon of Addiction

Addiction is defined as physiological or psychological dependence on exogenously administered substances. Addiction is an interplay between the brain's evolved reward system for adaptive behavior and the body's ability to detoxify ingested substances, evolved mainly through the competition between plants and animals as discussed in Chapter 8 (plants try to poison animals to keep from being eaten, and animals try to detoxify plants so that they can eat them). Chemicals that the brain produces under certain conditions attach to receptor molecules in brain cells and produce a physiological state that we perceive as pleasurable. Chemicals known as endogenous opioids[17] are produced by the hypothalamus, the hippocampus, and the midbrain when we are physically stressed and need relief from pain to accomplish activities potentially critical to our survival. For example, if we are seriously injured in an automobile accident, we are sometimes unaware of the pain of our injuries until after we have crawled up the embankment to get help. This neurochemical override of our normal pain response is adaptive because in situations of dire need we need to get ourselves out of immediate harm's way in order to survive. What happens in addiction is that outside drugs that mimic our brain chemicals are artificially administered to our systems, and they give us the same pain-free sensation. With enough use, our physiology becomes accommodated ("tolerant") to the drug, and we become dependent on it.

Where do the addictive drugs that wreak so much havoc in modern society come from? Plants, in their constant evolutionary experiments in biochemistry, have come up with a number of compounds that mimic our endogenous brain chemicals. What may kill an insect if it eats a plant may actually excite our brains because of the complex interactions of psychoactive chemicals and brain cell receptors. Heroin and its chemical relatives come from the poppy plant; cocaine comes from the coca plant; and cannabis comes from the marijuana plant. Like nicotine, discussed in Chapter 8, all of these chemicals are defenses that plants have evolved to protect themselves from being eaten by insects. Synthetic drugs like LSD (lysergic acid diethylamide) are merely human modifications of the basic plant chemical themes. Human attraction to and ability to metabolize ethyl alcohol (ethanol), also an addictive drug, may be almost as ancient as that to psychotropic drugs, but of a different adaptive function. R. Dudley has recently suggested that alcohol may have served as a cue to locating ripe or fermented fruit among our early primate frugivorous ancestors.[18] Alcohol may have first been used in primates as a food molecule, whereas the psychotropic drugs likely arose as plant toxins.

The exact biological and chemical interactions in our brain that underlie addiction are still being researched, but dopamine is an important component.[19] As mentioned above, dopamine is an R-complex chemical, produced in the substantia nigra, the midbrain, and the hypothalamus. It is a stimulatory or excitatory catecholamine (unlike serotonin, which is inhibitory). Its actions in the brain are integrated with those of epinephrine (adrenaline) in the basic physiological fight-or-flight response that accompanies danger. The mode of action of stimulatory drugs such as amphetamines and cocaine is to increase the amount of dopamine— amphetamines by stimulating its release from nerve cells, and cocaine by preventing its reuptake into nerve cells. Randolph Nesse and Kent Berridge have termed this system an evolved "liking" system, one that is rewarded when the drug is administered. They explain the continuing and spiraling use of addictive drugs even when they are no longer "liked" or enjoyed by the brain, by invoking a separate dopamine-dependent "wanting" system in the midbrain that promotes drug-seeking behavior. Whatever their exact evolutionary cause, these authors believe that "drugs of abuse create a signal in the brain that indicates, falsely, the arrival of a huge fitness benefit."[20]

Drugs and alcohol will undoubtedly loom large in the immediate human future. There is clear discordance between how we evolved to tolerate and/or use addictive substances in the past and how they have now become a major threat to our health. In the next chapter, we turn to some practical ways that we can use to render our evolved adaptations and current lives less discordant, and arrive at a closer approximation of psychological adaptive normality.

14

Uncivilized Solutions: Reestablishing Adaptive Normality in Your Life

Evolutionary biologist George Williams has written that in evolutionary medicine "adaptation is a more useful concept than normalcy."[1] Adaptation is, of course, central to understanding our biologically evolved nature,[2] but I believe that science can and should provide medicine with a reliable description of human biological normality. Indeed, both adaptation and "normalcy" have evolved, and it is best to view both as intrinsic parts of human biology. There is such a thing as the "wisdom of the body," a term coined by the great cardiac physiologist Frank Starling in the 1930s, and evolution alone explains how such bodily wisdom came about.

This chapter includes a number of recommendations about preserving your health and preventing illnesses that are derived from human evolutionary principles, as discussed in previous chapters. Some of the recommendations may seem unconventional and unusual from the limited perspective of one culture and one time. But they are strongly indicated by human evolutionary history, which encompasses all cultures and spans eons. Nevertheless, further research and clinical experience may well serve to modify them in the future, and you should consult your physician when applying these principles to your own unique situation.

Optimal Human Diet

People in the industrialized world today eat only half the volume of food by weight that even our recent ancestors ate, yet they are at least 15 percent heavier for the same height.[3] We should be eating more, not less, to lose weight, decreasing our energy:satiety index (chapter 12). The issue is, eat what?

We have been dietary generalists—omnivores—since the ape-human divergence. Because we have been eating a great deal of animal protein for over 2 million years, it makes evolutionary sense to keep meat in our diet. Because we have been eating a wide variety of plant foods for an even longer period of time, we should adjust our fruit and vegetable intake to reflect this variety. Because fibrous foods formed a major part of our diet in the past, we should include these in similar quantities in our diet now. The only caveats to these conclusions are that the intrinsic nature of the food, such as meat or fiber, may have changed over the millennia, and we need to ensure that what we are eating has not been subject to modern modifications.

Well-established precepts lead to a high-protein, high-fiber, and high-plant/fruit diet. Table 7 gives the guidelines for a diet consistent with the broad tenets of human evolution. As discussed in earlier chapters, this diet will help to prevent such conditions as diverticulosis, appendicitis, ulcerative colitis, and colon cancers. Low overall calories help you to reduce the proportion of stored fat in your body. Low salt content cuts down your chances of developing high blood pressure and heart disease. A moderate amount of muscle tissue and animal fat (meat) in such a paleodiet provides you with important protein and high-density lipoproteins (HDLs) necessary for keeping your cell membranes, blood vessels, skin, and nervous system well-nourished and well-maintained. Lots of fruit and vegetables gives you high but evolutionarily normal amounts of vitamins A, B complex, C, D, and K.

Table 7. Paleodiet Guidelines

Goal	Solution
Avoid dietary carcinogens, mutagens, and teratogens	Choose organic and natural foods whenever possible; moderate alcohol intake; no psychotropic drugs; no tobacco use; monitor environmental and occupational exposure to toxins—e.g., lead paint, air pollution, dust, and volatile fumes
High fiber content of food (30–50 grams per day)	Eat fruits, with the peel, rather than drinking fruit juice; eat tubers, such as potatoes and yams, with the skin; eat insect chitin; eat nuts; avoid grains and cereals
High protein content of food (constituting approximately 30 percent of daily energy)	Eat lean animal muscle and organ meats, preferable from free-range animals, such as chickens, bison, and deer; eat eggs, again preferably from free-range chickens; eat high protein vegetables, such as soy; eat insects
Fat content of food constituting 20–25 percent of daily energy	Eat meat with moderate fat content—e.g., bacon; eat plant foods with high highly unsaturated fatty acid content
Low salt content of food and high potassium-sodium ratio	Eat fresh, unsalted foods; avoid canned foods; avoid soft drinks and carbonated beverages; eat very few potato chips
Very low refined sugar content of food	Eat honey and naturally sweet foods, such as fruits, and avoid all sugars, including artificial sweeteners; give up soft drinks
High content of antioxidants	Eat foods with high vitamin C, such as citrus fruits, and high vitamin A, such as spinach
High content of calcium	Eat yogurt and drink skim milk, if not lactose intolerant; eat bones; eat insects
Variable diet	Eat different things each day; do not take megadoses of any dietary supplements or vitamins; gorge on one preferred food each month—e.g., dates
Low cereal grain content of food	Grains should constitute a low proportion of diet and should be whole grain

Debates about the optimal human diet continue to rage. Many preventive physicians and nutritionists fervently believe in the benefits of a purely vegetarian diet, supplemented with concentrated forms of vitamins and nutrients that your body is not getting from meat. The Physicians Committee for Responsible Medicine, a nonprofit preventive medicine group, advocates a vegetarian diet,[4] and vegetarian nutritionist Marion Nestle recently has gone so far as to question the paleoanthropological evidence for meat eating.[5] Our best evidence, however, just does not support the argument that a vegetarian diet—that is, a diet composed of fruits, legumes, seeds, and other plants to the exclusion to animal protein—is the ideal, "natural" one for the human species. Hominid dental and jaw anatomy—the large molar teeth, massive jaws, and huge chewing muscles of australopithecines and early *Homo*—make more sense as adaptations to omnivorous diets of tough foods, including meat, rather than vegetarian specializations. In our early primate evolutionary history, as plesiadapiforms (Level 11) and prosimians (Level 12), it is true that a substantial component of the diet was made up of vegetation, but at the same time the teeth of these primate ancestors indicate that they were insectivorous, deriving substantial animal protein from invertebrates. Analysis of isotopic composition of tooth enamel shows that 3 million years ago, South African australopithecines "ate not only fruits and leaves but also ... high-quality animal foods."[6] Recently discovered bone tools in South Africa show that some 2.5 million years ago, early hominids habitually dug up termite mounds for food.[7] Abundant animal bones with unambiguous stone tool cut marks dated to after 2.6 million years ago attest to the antiquity of meat eating as well.

Most of the recommendations in Table 7 follow directly from the various discussions in prior chapters, but there are a few innovations of the natural diet recommended here that set it apart from some other paleodiets.

The recommendation for natural and organic food sources is, whenever possible, based on the effects of carcinogenic, mutagenic, and teratogenic effects of insecticides, synthetic fertilizers, and antibiotics used in agriculture and animal husbandry. Evidence of these effects is still arguable in some experts' minds. Yet insects are far more closely related to us than are plants, and it makes evolutionary sense to deduce that a substance that poisons insects, but not plants, could also likely poison us. Organic and natural produce is the safest, but if you must eat standard supermarket fruits and vegetables, at least wash them off thoroughly.

The international hoopla over genetically modified food plants has turned what appeared to be a benign use of genetics into a threat to our global food resources. Is the public resistance to genetically modified plants simply because most people do not understand the technology, or is their stubborn refusal to accept this new type of plant food akin to the publics' opposition to nuclear power plants in America—based on real danger despite the experts' assurances? Genetic modification promises the advantage of conferring resistance to plants that lessens or obviates the need for the use of pesticides. However, "genetic resistance" may translate to the plant producing its own intrinsic insecticide, potentially just as injurious to humans.[8] In assessing whether genetically modified plants are safe, the bottom line would seem to be answering the question of how they interact biologically with other life-forms, including humans. All too often, people make the mistake of thinking that they are apart from nature, not a part of nature, and an evolutionary perspective is critical in counteracting this notion. A reasonable question to ask is "If a plant strain is not palatable to insects, why is it not palatable, and why should people eat it?"

Hormones fed to food animals to make them grow larger are a potential cause of concern because they can promote hormonally dependent cancers. However, the concentrations of remnant hormones in meat is so low that biological effects seem to be minimal. Nevertheless, meat is only one component of our overall diet, and its hormone content contributes to the dosage effect of exogenous chemicals that we now ingest. Better to go for free-range chickens and hormone-free beef and similar sources of animal protein, if you can get them.

The real toxicity in commercially bought meat is its fat content. Fat tastes good, and "marbling" (streaks of fat within the muscle fibers) in steaks has been selected in beef cattle for decades. Lamb, mutton, and pork are also esteemed because of their fat content. Lean red meats like venison, bison, ostrich, rabbit, squirrel, or turtle are excellent low-fat alternatives to standard meats. Fish is an excellent source of lean meat. Obtaining some of these foods takes forethought, but in addition to making your diet healthier, they just might liven up your cuisine. You can now buy most alternative meats online or by mail order, or you can hunt them down yourself.

Hunting and Gathering in the Modern World

Variety was a key element of ancient hominid diets—not only for plant foods, but also for sources of animal protein. We should get over our recent historical focus on only a few food species (cow, chicken, pig, and various fish) and diversify. All animal muscle is equivalent, and the feeling that some species are inappropriate for human consumption—such as rats—is nothing more than prejudice. Rats in fact eat much the same diet as we do (that's why they live so well close to humans), and their meat is perfectly safe to eat. International cuisines from Chinese to French siege cuisine have incorporated rats, and even the U.S. Peace Corps cookbook, *Where There Is No McDonalds'*, has a recipe for "rats in the mood." You can also eat the bones of small animals—a usual custom in Africa and an excellent source of calcium.

Catching and eating a rat may not end up being the next food craze in America (although it was required fare in the first series of *Survivor*). There is indeed a stigma attached to rats. So if you feel more comfortable eating game bagged in the great outdoors, one solution is to fish, hunt, and trap it yourself—traditionally highly valued, primarily male (but not necessarily so) pursuits, and a good source of exercise. Another source is scavenging—also an ancestral hominid pursuit, even more ancient than hunting. One good place for modern-day scavenging is the highway, and the *Road Kill Cookbook*[9] provides a number of excellent dishes to be made from the various species to be found. Fresh roadkills are the most palatable. Opossum stuffed with sweet potato is my favorite. Of course, skulking by the roadside for dead animals may seem too undignified for you; if so, there are many mail-order sources for broadening your dietary choices. Some web sites are provided at the end of this chapter.

Even more challenging to entrenched dietary customs is expanding our choices outside vertebrates. The Harvard University Faculty Club, for example, daringly has horse on its menu, left over from World War II belt-tightening, but there are no dishes made from terrestrial invertebrates. The Explorers Club Annual Banquet, featuring such exotic food choices as hippo and even a bit of frozen extinct Siberian mammoth, did go so far once as to offer an insect-only menu, cosponsored with a society of entomologists. Insects are an abundant and excellent source of protein, calcium, and fiber, they require much less feed and are thus more ecologically efficient sources of protein than standard beef or chicken, they are low fat, and you can eat common garden pests, thus reducing the need for pesticides. They fit into our dietary repertoire at Levels 11 and 12, a period of about 17 million years of our evolution.

Eating insects is really not all that unthinkable. Aquatic invertebrates, such as shrimp, crab, and lobster, are closely related to insects, and entire restaurant chains specializing in one or more of these types of seafood flourish. Escargot, those mushy-bodied mollusks also related to insects and known more commonly as "snails," have been a charter member of haute cuisine for centuries. And we already unwittingly ingest a fair number of insects. For example, regulations of the U.S. Food and Drug Administration allow as many as 56 insect parts in a unit of peanut butter, up to 60 aphids in 31.5 ounces of frozen broccoli, and up to 3 fruit-fly maggots per 200 grams of tomato juice.[10] In choosing insects for your cuisine, evolutionary principles are quite important to remember, however. Warning coloration of certain species can indicate poisons or noxious taste. Insectivore (or "entomophage") author David Gordon suggests the following rule of thumb: "Red, orange or yellow, forgo this small fellow. Black, green or brown, go ahead and toss him down."[11] Mexican entomologist Julieta Ramos-Elorduy also provides a number of excellent recipes for insects.[12]

The variety of plants eaten by hunter-gatherers is astounding to us moderns, who live on a boring menu of about 10 or 20 species, all provided by agriculture. Ethnographic accounts show that technologically primitive peoples know, collect, and eat hundreds of varieties of plants throughout the seasonal rounds of the year. Ignorance of what species might be edible and collectible in our backyards prevents many of us from eating a wider diversity of wild plants. And it is always possible to grow your own.

Not only does our choice of foods unduly restrict the variety of our diet, so do our social patterns of eating. This can become unhealthy. Sitting down and eating three meals a day is not the evolutionarily ancient way of eating. We either snacked most of the day as eatables became available, or we gorged to excess when we were hungry and managed to find a major source of food all at once. One can imagine a fruiting date palm or a downed antelope. Snacks when you are working are a great idea, but make them low-carbohydrate snacks—fruits, carrots, pemmican, seeds, or unsalted nuts. Eating small meals and frequent snacking is a standard medical recommendation for patients with peptic ulcer and other gastrointestinal disorders, but it is not a bad idea for all of us. This is not a recommendation to give up sit-down meals, which are some of the few times that Western families ever see one another. Rather, have meals that offer variety and that have vitamins and bulk, but not a lot of calories.

Gorging has been traditionally frowned upon in our culture. It is considered to be an indication of uncontrolled desire and gluttony, but it is certainly a part of our evolutionary heritage. In the past, however, occasional gorging was always accompanied by significant periods of fasting, simply because of the nature of food resources. As discussed in chapter 13, this aspect of our digestive physiology is not unreasonably part of the etiology of bulimia—a condition in which forced vomiting replaces the natural lack of food that would follow a food binge. Gorging every once in a while can assist materially in the abatement of cravings. It is best to gorge on something that is healthy and that you like. I like dates, for example, and I tend to get a package of them and eat them all at once. Then I don't eat them for again for several months. Although not fully tested, controlled gorging may be a treatment for overeating certain foods. For example, it may be better to gorge on Moon Pies or Twinkies for a period sufficient to get sick of them for life, and then return to a normal diet. Conversely, not eating—short-term fasting—fits well with the normal Paleolithic rhythm and offsets any positive net calorie gain from occasional gorging.

Honey, Milk, Alcohol, and Our Daily Bread

Sugar is not a food on which to gorge. Yet, by one estimate, Americans eat their own weight in sugar each year (if they weigh 120 pounds). Sugar is clearly contributory to diabetes and is a major cause of obesity. Why do people like to eat sweet things covered with sugar?

The antiquity of our sweet tooth goes back to the early primates and their diet of forest fruits, full of the sugar fructose (Level 11 and 12 adaptations). At the hominid level, we have an anciently evolved relationship with honey, documented by the behavior of the African honey bird (or honeyguide). This relative of the woodpecker has evolved to lead hominids as well as African honey badgers to bees' nests. While on safari in Kenya, Theodore Roosevelt observed honey birds chattering loudly and then invariably leading his men to honey.[13] Modern African honey hunters still follow these birds to the trees in which bees' nests are found, rob the bees of their honey, and leave some honeycomb for the bird. Honeyguides have a uniquely adapted gut bacterial flora that can break down beeswax. Their take from the beehive thus is neatly ecologically partitioned from the honey that their partners, the humans or the honey badgers, take home. If the bird tried to get the honey itself, the bees would sting it to death (even though honeyguides have very thick skin). How ancient this coevolved adaptation may be is anybody's guess, but for such well-established behaviors and physiologies to have evolved suggests at least hundreds of thousands if not millions of years. Although ancient, our acquisition of honey was seasonal, and nowhere near the amount of sugar that we now eat.

Sweet fruits have undoubtedly been on the primate menu for many millions of years. Naturally occurring sugars then are adaptively the best for inclusion in our diet. Most of the carbohydrates that nonhuman primates and hunter-gatherer humans eat come from fruit and other plant sources. Refined sugars and artificial sugars are evolutionary neologisms and should be avoided.

Dairy products came into the human culinary world too late in evolution to be considered part of our natural and normal diet, according to Boyd Eaton and colleagues.[14] For many populations around the world this may be true, but for some people who have evolved the enzymes to digest lactose, the sugar in milk, dairy products are not only tolerated, they are important dietary constituents. Human evolution did not stop 10,000 years ago, and there are significant changes within Level 17, taken to begin at 40,000 years ago. The variation seen within populations (some individuals even within a lactase-positive population may not have the enzyme) and the evolutionary history of each population need to be taken into consideration when promoting optimal diets. For peoples who have descended from thousands of generations of herders, widespread in Eurasia and parts of Africa, lactase is an enzyme that has been maintained from infancy into adulthood and allows milk to be digested. Partially fermented milk in the form of bacterially degraded yogurt and cheeses is more easily digested, but raw milk is quite compatible with the evolved capabilities of these people and should not be excluded from their diets. The elderly, particularly, can benefit from the calcium and vitamin D in milk, which helps to prevent osteoporosis (thin bones).

The enzymes for breaking down alcohol, primarily alcohol dehydrogenase, are also present in our livers, and attest to the fact that we can safely imbibe and digest small amounts of ethyl alcohol (ethanol)—about the same amount as might naturally occur in fermented fruit.[15] A paleodiet thus does not have to be an alcohol-free diet, and, indeed, moderate intakes of alcohol have been shown to have positive effects on health. But drinking more than the equivalent of a glass or two of wine with meals is too much. Some populations, such as many in Asia, have low levels of alcohol dehydrogenase, and thus low tolerances for alcohol.

Various grasses were brought under domestication worldwide beginning about 10,000 years ago. These species include barley, millet, wheat, and rye in the Middle East, teff in northeastern Africa, rice in eastern Asia, corn in Central America, and quinoa in northwestern South America. These new grains as major components of diet undoubtedly had significant effects on the gastrointestinal physiology of the populations which began to eat them. Populations had to evolve to tolerate them and their toxins. As discussed in chapter 12, some specific gastrointestinal diseases are related to remaining immunological reactions to these recently introduced plant foods.

Some of the same populations that evolved the ability to digest milk sugar, for example, tend to have allergic reactions to the covering of wheat grains ("gluten"). The gastrointestinal condition known as "celiac sprue" results. Grain-based agriculture in many northern European populations was just not a major source of food until relatively recently, and evolution did not select out the primitive reaction of IgE immune response to plant proteins.

Vitamins and Minerals

There are some 13 chemical compounds recognized as "vitamins": the 8 B-complex vitamins and vitamin C (all water soluble), and the fat-soluble vitamins A, D, E, and K. A widely used medical biochemistry dictionary defines a vitamin as "an organic substance that is distributed in food stuffs in minute amounts and is needed for normal nutrition of the organism."[16] Essential minerals are the inorganic (non-carbon-based) elements that the body needs. Their roles in the body are all surprisingly ancient, having evolved in the earliest single-celled organisms. The B complex vitamins evolved at Level 2 as catalysts in metabolism, especially in the transfer of energy, and they are essential to all cellular organisms. Vitamin C is necessary for the formation of collagen, the basic structural protein of organisms' bodies. All these vitamins dissolve in water, are not stored in the body, and are excreted in the urine. Vitamin C utilization in primates has a unique evolutionary history, and we will return to it in the following section.

The fat-soluble vitamins probably evolved later than the water-soluble vitamins because their functions are generally targeted for more advanced animal structures and functions. Vitamin A derivatives, for example, have a profound effect on animal developmental patterns, such as the limb bud of a chick or the tail of a salamander.[17] As further proof of vitamin A's time of origin, it is known to be important in the formation of visual pigments in the retina of the eye, another Level 5 adaptation.[18]

Vitamin K may similarly have evolved at the earliest animal stage of our evolution from a precursor molecule similar to one still found in bacteria. Its function is closely tied to the clotting of blood. The blood clotting system is a cascade of interactions evolved prior to the split of vertebrates and invertebrates, again a Level 5 adaptation.[19]

Vitamin E may be the most primitive of the fat-soluble vitamins. It is concerned with scavenging oxygen free radicals and maintaining cell membranes. Its evolution may date to the first aerobic organisms at Level 2.

Vitamin D is likely the most recently evolved vitamin, dating to the time of the first vertebrates (Level 7). Vitamin D has a major role in maintaining cells' levels of calcium, critical for bone development. It is produced in the skin by ultraviolet-B radiation from the Sun, and it has undergone major evolutionary change among hominids (Levels 15 through 17; see pages 37–39).

Vitamins are one of the most commonly ingested dietary supplements, and fantastic claims are made for their presumed therapeutic benefits. A standard statement is "Vitamins—Our bodies cannot get enough from food."[20] Yet most medical knowledge of vitamins is limited to their deficiency states—what happens when we don't get enough vitamins. An evolutionary perspective can help us in understanding what normal levels of vitamins in our bodies should be.

A little bit of medicine may work wonders, so shouldn't a lot be even better? Unfortunately, this logic, though linear, does not work. An old African missionary doctor once told me about a rural patient who was brought to his clinic suffering from an acute malarial attack. He gave the man a loading dose of quinine, and since he lived far away, an additional three weeks' supply. But the man returned the very next day, his malaria much better but with a terrible headache, abdominal pain, and ringing in his ears. He had taken all the quinine, using the rationale that the first dose made him feel so much better, the rest would make him feel better still.

Like quinine, vitamins and minerals show the phenomenon of hormesis—positive effects at low dosages and negative health effects at high dosages.[21] Natural selection has acted to calibrate the levels of nutrients needed in our bodies to our diet, and of course there were no vitamin pills in the Plio-Pleistocene. So latter-day arguments for megadoses of vitamins, claiming that our "natural diet" cannot meet nutritional needs, are largely fanciful.

In some few cases, vitamin supplements may make evolutionary sense in circumstances significantly changed from ancestral environments.

Vitamin C, Primate Energy, and Antioxidants

Undoubtedly the most prominent vitamin enthusiast in recent years was the two-time Nobel laureate Linus Pauling. Pauling believed that the antioxidant properties of vitamin C (ascorbate) could prevent a number of maladies—from the common cold to cancer.[22] He recommended massive daily dosages, around 10,000 milligrams, and followed his own advice. Pauling died in 1994 at the age of 93, of prostate cancer, so the large amounts of vitamin C probably didn't kill him. However, in such elevated amounts, they probably didn't do him very much good, either. Vitamin C is a water-soluble vitamin, so what the body does not need, it excretes. But excessive vitamin C can cause mouth ulcers, diarrhea, flatulence, light-headedness during exertion, and can even reverse its antioxidant properties.[23]

In the physiology of animals, ascorbate plays a central role in the synthesis of collagen, a basic structural constituent of the extracellular matrix (the space between cells in the body). Paul Morris emphasized the importance of the extracellular matrix in development as a shared characteristic of all animals.[24] It is a Level 4 or 5 adaptation and dates back at least a billion years. If the amount of ascorbate in the body is low, collagen fails to develop properly and the deficiency disease scurvy results. Scurvy causes bone and muscle weakness, internal bleeding, skin lesions, and loss of teeth. The disease cannot afflict most animals because they possess the four enzymes necessary to convert glucose to ascorbic acid.[25] However, endogenous production of ascorbate does take energy and uses up glucose in the body.

The primate ancestors of humans lost the ascorbate-forming enzyme, L-gulonolactone oxidase, because of a mutation some 45 million years ago, after the divergence of the lemurs and lorises and before the divergence of the tarsiers and anthropoid primates (Level 12).[26] Their largely frugivorous diet provided abundant sources of the vitamin, relaxing natural selection for endogenous production of ascorbate. The mutation that knocked out L-gulonolactone oxidase allowed the precursor of ascorbate, gulonolactone, to accumulate. Excess gulonolactone, following one of its alternate metabolic pathways, served as a precursor to pentose sugars that could then enter the metabolic pathway, providing glucose, glycogen (its stored form), and extra energy. Higher primates traded in an ancient pathway used for maintaining the body's extracellular matrix and made redundant because of dietary changes, and exchanged it for a new, higher-energy storage pathway. Given the changing environments of the late Paleocene, when forests and food sources were shrinking, this evolutionary scenario makes sense. It also jibes with the observation that other high-metabolism animals like certain birds, bats, and fast-swimming fish independently lost the enzyme for forming ascorbate.

What does this evolutionary perspective tell us about modern human requirements for vitamin C? First, baseline levels of vitamin C should not be more than our prosimian ancestors produced before the L-gulonolactone oxidase gene mutated. Estimates of this amount are in the range of 500 to 600 milligrams per day. The amount of vitamin C taken in by hunter-gatherers is in the same range. This amount is more than the recommended daily amount to prevent scurvy, but substantially below the megadoses advocated by Linus Pauling and others. Only if oxidative assaults are severe, as in burn patients, should massive amounts of vitamin C be taken.

Vitamin B$_{12}$ and Chronic Fatigue Syndrome

The B-complex vitamins evolved at Level 2 primarily as catalysts for metabolism, especially in the transfer of energy. Like vitamin C, they are water soluble and are not stored in the body. Most vitamin B requirements are met by a normal natural diet, as suggested here. Deficiencies of the B vitamins are rare, but vitamin B$_{12}$ deficiency is a danger for strict vegetarians.

Vitamin B$_{12}$, however, is also being used as a therapy for chronic fatigue syndrome (CFS), a disease of civilization that is, like fibromyalgia (chapter 11), of obscure causation. Biochemist Martin Pall has suggested that physical stress from infection, trauma, chemical exposure, and even psychological stress cause the cellular release of nitric oxide.[27] This stimulus then sets in motion several biochemical feedback loops that increase the levels of peroxynitrite, a powerful oxidant in the body that damages tissues and kills mitochondria. The mitochondria are the energy-producing organelles within cells, and their loss leads to chronic fatigue. Vitamin B_{12} in the form of hydroxocobalamin can act as a nitric oxide scavenger and thus potentially break the vicious cycles of CFS. In an environment of increased stress, increased levels of Vitamin B_{12} may well be adaptive.

Vitamin E, Heart Disease, and Cancers

Vitamin E, also known as tocopherol, is a close second to vitamin C as the dietary supplement most often taken by Americans. Vitamin E acts as an antioxidant, and several studies in the 1990s indicated that it helped to prevent the cellular oxidative damage that underlies arterial wall damage, the onset of cancers, cataracts, and even Alzheimer's disease. But follow-up clinical trails have been less than conclusive.

Work by S. Christen and colleagues showed that the most effective antioxidant form of vitamin E, the kind in our normal diet, is gamma-tocopherol.[28] The major kind of vitamin E put into vitamin supplements is alpha-tocopherol, a different form of the vitamin, thus possibly explaining the conflicting clinical results. Gamma-tocopherol scavenges peroxynitrite, whose destructive actions are hypothesized to lead to arterial lining damage and cancer.

The value of vitamin E in the modern world lies in its ability to scavenge oxidants in our bodies, deriving from such sources as nitric oxide in air pollution. Vitamin E levels in hunter-gatherers and wild-living, nonhuman primate species are not accurately known, but an argument could be made that somewhat higher levels than those seen in the natural state might be warranted in modern polluted circumstances. Vitamin E in the average American diet was found to be adequate (about 15 milligrams for adults and 19 milligrams for nursing mothers) by a 2000 survey conducted by the U.S. Institute of Medicine,[29] suggesting that dietary sources, particularly oils and nuts, meet physiological demands. If taken as a supplement, Vitamin E, although it is stored in fat, does not lead to a recognized overdosage condition.

Vitamin D, Rickets, Melanoma, and Acne

The dark pigment, melanin, may be the earliest antioxidant to have evolved.[30] It is a "solid-state" antioxidant found in the skin and the retina, where it quenches free radicals formed by sunlight, and in parts of the brain, such as the substantia nigra, where it possibly serves to prevent oxidative damage to the well-oxygenated brain. Vitamin D is produced in the skin, and it is essential for calcium metabolism and bone production. In hominid evolution, there was an interplay between the antioxidant effects of melanin and the production of vitamin D in the skin.

The original skin color of the first hominids may have been white, with a coat of black hair (like the chimpanzee), black with a coat of black hair (like the gorilla), or black and largely hairless. When hominids lost their coat of hair, it is certain that their skin was darkly melanic, like all tropical human populations today. Dark skin blocks ultraviolet radiation and thus prevents sunburn. Melanin also absorbs free radicals produced by the same radiation that could damage the skin and the structures within it, such as sweat glands. Enough ultraviolet radiation gets through the skin to produce vitamin D in the dermis layer of skin.[31]

When hominids left the African tropics and colonized higher latitudes, sunlight intensity was significantly lower during the winter months, during which darkly pigmented skin did not allow sufficient UV radiation to penetrate the skin to make adequate amounts of vitamin D. The deficiency disease rickets resulted. In the primitive state, rickets would have been a fatal or near-fatal disease because bones are left so weak and malformed that walking is impossible. A recent suggestion by N. G. Jablonski and G. Chaplin is that pigmented skin also protected blood levels of the vitamin folate (a B-complex vitamin subject to rapid denaturation by sunlight) from being diminished.[32] A lack of folate during pregnancy leads to severe birth defects affecting the neural tube, such as spina bifida. Darkly pigmented individuals living in high latitudes would have been severely dealt with by natural selection. Dark skin evolved to light skin rapidly in these populations.

When modern humans whose Level 17 ancestors evolved in a tropical part of the world relocate to a significantly higher or lower latitude, vitamin D supplements may well be warranted, to prevent rickets. When light-skinned humans relocate to tropical locations, care needs to be taken to avoid skin damage by intense sunlight, known to be an inducer of skin cancers, including melanoma. Although not generally recognized as a requirement, folate levels in the diets of these individuals should be high.

Anecdotal, but potentially valid nonetheless, is the apparent higher incidence of acne in light-skinned populations, correlated with high androgen hormone levels. Acne seems to be caused by free radical oxidants in the skin, and when severe is treated by retinoic acid (a variety of vitamin A). Melanin may act as a free radical scavenger in darkly pigmented skin, thus staving off the inflammations of acne. If correct, this model would argue for acne being a Level 16 or 17 affliction and a by-product of natural selection for vitamin D absorption in high-latitude populations.

Iron, Anemia, and Hemochromatosis

Iron is the atom at the center of the heme molecule, the molecular building block of blood. The body needs a lot of iron when it is making blood. But iron is also a mineral that bacteria need to reproduce, so one primitive antibacterial strategy used by the body is to sequester iron—lock it away from invading bacteria.[33]

The hereditary disease "hemochromatosis" results from too much iron in the body, leading to liver, heart, and neurological problems. It is X-linked, thus affecting men more frequently than women, and is more common in European populations. The condition is treated by phlebotomy—bleeding a patient. The evolutionary medicine of this disease has been elusive, although its incidence primarily in one population, Europeans, argues for it to be a recent evolutionary event (Level 17). One explanation is that greater bonding of iron was needed by individuals adapting to agriculture and a substantially lower amount of meat in the diet. But this idea runs counter to the observation that Europeans seem to be one of the last populations to have made the transition to grains, as witnessed by the high incidence of celiac sprue. A more likely hypothesis is that hemochromatosis is an adaptation to chronic blood loss and the attendant anemia. Menstruation can lead to anemia in modern women, but this does not explain the high incidence of hemochromatosis in one population, or the presence of the trait preferentially in males. Chronic blood loss through parasitic infection, especially by hookworm (or other similar helminthic parasites), may be the underlying condition that the high retention rate of iron in hemochromatosis helped to counteract. These parasites currently infect about a fifth of the world's population—about a billion people.[34] Adult worms lodge in the intestines, and each ingest about 0.25 millilitre of blood per day.[35] An infection of 500 worms can cause an estimated loss of over a liter of blood a day, and significant anemia. The ability to retain iron in hemochromatosis would be a significant advantage to an individual living with high hookworm infestation. Modern treatment includes close monitoring of iron levels in the body and phlebotomy (or frequent blood donations).

Fitness and Strength

The term for physiological resilience and anatomical robustness—"fitness"—is the same as the technical term for a trait or an adaptation favored by natural selection. The 19th-century social scientist Herbert Spencer first coined the phrase "survival of the fittest" to describe Darwin's new theory, and its message can be applied in a different sense to modern life. "Physical fitness," as the term is colloquially used, is an acquired character, built up by regular activity and behavior. "Fitness" as used by evolutionary biologists is an intrinsic trait of a gene as played out in the development and biology of an organism. The two concepts are related but quite distinct. In an evolutionarily normal world, evolutionary fitness assumes physical fitness. When this assumption is not met, we have a situation that we have termed "discordance"—the main cause of the diseases of civilization.

For most of us, our jobs keep us inside and immobile for most of our day. And when we finish work, we usually have a hundred things to do, our family is waiting for us, or we are too tired. What can you do to get back onto an evolutionarily normal pattern of physical activity?

Unfortunately, we are adapted to be lazy, but this adaptation for laziness makes evolutionary sense. When there is no pressing need, we just do not jump up and decide to run five miles. If we have enough food, if there is no immediate danger, and if we have a comfortable place to sit, we tend to stay just where we are. Hypoactivity when there are no physiological or environmental calls to action conserves energy and reduces chances for injury and trauma. What is unusual about our modern situation is that those calls to action never come. So we have to contrive them, with due deference to evolved adaptations.

Exercise, first of all, needs to be regular. Our R-complex needs to become accustomed to doing exercise every day. Secondly, we need to tie exercise into our daily food quest. Make a pact with yourself that to eat you must exercise—a mile on the exercise bike for lunch. Chase down that tuna sandwich. This sounds funny, but it ties in exercise with your limbic system, and you associate a negative physiological stimulus (hunger) with activity, which is a normal evolved response, and then you associate exercise with the positive reward of eating. Finally, your neocortex can be brought in to help support your exercise plan by recognizing how much more mental productivity you have, how much better you feel, and how much better you look.

Exercise can also be designed into your food quest. Gardening can be good exercise and also yields excellent fresh vegetables, which you can grow without pesticides or fertilizers. Gathering can be done at commercial farms where you can pick your own apples, berries, or other produce. If you hunt, trap, or fish for food, make sure that you do it the Paleolithic way—lots of walking, and no firearms. Using a bow and arrow is a fairly advanced hunting (and fishing) technique, but primitive, Kalahari bushman–style bows and arrows can be ordered over the Internet. Hunting with spears, launched either by hand or by atlatls (throwing sticks), is great exercise. The World Atlatl Association now has a website (www.worldatlatl.org) for more information. Or you could hunt the way some South American aboriginal people did—without weapons—just by running relays until a pursued animal is too exhausted to run away anymore. This is a particularly good way to hunt if you would rather let the animal go and then stop by the supermarket on your way home.

Adaptively Normal Exercise

There is no question that humans are anatomically and physiologically adapted to active modes of life. We sweat, from largely hairless skin, to dissipate heat from burning calories. Our skeletal muscles have the capability to develop more energy-producing mitochondria and to increase the size of the cells over time as we exercise them. Our hearts respond to increased workloads by pumping more blood with each contraction. As our joints move, our ligaments stay stretched and flexible. Our bones stay strong as they resist the forces of gravity and muscular tension. We saw in chapter 9 that regular physical activity causes insulin receptors in muscles to increase in number so that glucose can be taken in efficiently and burned. Exercise also lowers cholesterol levels in the blood.

The fossil and archaeological record of ancient humans, filled in with ethnographic detail gathered from modern hunters and gatherers, informs us of our adaptively normal pattern of activity. Daily life in the past required both endurance fitness, as in running down prey or walking long distances to gather food, and strength, as in thrusting a spear into an attacking cave bear or carrying a heavy load of wood or food for several miles. Our daily routines now depend on laborsaving machines and conveniences that obviate the necessity of all but the most feeble muscular effort on our part. They were invented and built by hominids in whom laziness evolved as an important counterbalance to industry. Hunters and gatherers all take abundant time off to recuperate from the rigors of the hunt or the forage. But to actually escape regular physical exertion—to the extent of causing disease—was not an eventuality that the inventors of the automobile, the remote control, the microwave oven, and the Big Mac ever anticipated, if they thought about it at all.

Most Americans are way out of the zone of adaptively normal exercise. But if physical exertion is so much a part of our heritage and so important to our health, how could this have happened? To add to this conundrum, people *like* to exercise. We call this fun and games, or sports. Why would people *not* want to do this?

It is beyond the scope of this book to delve into the social psychology of modern Western sedentism, but certainly the press of time constraints is the most common excuse for being too preoccupied to be able to engage in physical exercise. What about all the time that was supposed to be saved by those "laborsaving" devices? Where did it go and what is it used for? Recent surveys by the AC Nielsen Company show that the average American watches 3 hours and 43 minutes of television a day.[36] That's certainly a significant part of the answer. And could it be that such a laborsaving device as the automobile actually takes up much more of our time than it saves? Married mothers with school-age children spend an average 66 minutes a day driving—that is almost 17 solid days a year in the car.[37] Maybe it would be a good idea to get Justin and Heather to walk to soccer practice, along with Mom, instead of piling into the SUV.

Another part of the underlying rationale for ignoring physical activity is that mainstay of the American Way, the Puritan Ethic. Physical exercise was fine so long as it was "work." But to "play" was a waste of time if it did not make you any money, vain if you were doing it to look better, and probably sinful if you were doing it to feel better. Don't get me wrong. I was educated in part by New England Puritans, some of the best, and I appreciate their good qualities. But even today, we call exercising a "workout" to exorcise the demons of our Puritan forebears.

Play is the evolutionarily adapted way to get more exercise. Prehistoric exercise was episodic, varied, socially integrated, and different from season to season. Your exercise should be as well. The work approach to fitness—assembly-line machines in an exercise club day after day—should be avoided. It's boring, and it's difficult to keep up. Use machines and free weights for strength, but vary what you do day to day, using different muscle groups and different routines. Intersperse "playouts" with endurance exercises like jogging, walking, and aerobics, or playing sports such as tennis, racquetball, or basketball (with your spouse, friends, kids, or people you work with). Boyd Eaton and Colleagues also emphasize the importance of flexibility as a third component of fitness (along with strength and endurance). Use warm-ups, stretching, and cooldowns to build up to and taper off from vigorous activity without causing muscle pulls, tendon strains, ligament tears, and heart arrhythmias. The benefits of fluidity of movement and the lack of many aches and pains, even into your 70s and 80s and beyond, will be significant. An effective paleo-exercise program is attainable and fun. But you must take the hour or so out of your day to do it—frequently the most difficult habit to get into.

Stress Avoidance

What an enigmatic situation we modern humans find ourselves in! Few real dangers, but riddled by worry, anxiety, and stress. Psychological stress for most people comes from the social contract—what they are expected to do, what they have promised to do, what social and legal norms prescribe for them, getting what family and society owe them, and keeping up social appearances. Financial concerns are near the top of the list of stressors.

Emotional stress has some similarities to physical stress, but also some important differences. Our adrenergic system begins to produce epinephrine (adrenaline) in anticipation of a coming confrontation, be it an attacking cave bear or an impending presentation at a board meeting. If we survive the cave-bear attack, we usually need the steroids and endogenous opioids that our body produces in order to recuperate from our physical exertion and wounds. If we survive the board meeting, we are relieved, but we may be left shaking with excess epinephrine. There has been no physical release, no real emotional conclusion, and no endorphins to make ourselves feel better. Civilization is just too far from our evolutionary roots. What is the solution?

Emotional support from family and friends, open discussion about problems at work or school, seeking fair hearings over grievances, displacement of feelings of pent-up aggression ("blowing off steam"), and sometimes even direct confrontations with difficult people will help to relieve stress. When all else fails, nonhuman primates and many human cultures around the world use trial by combat. Physical fighting has long been eschewed in most legal systems as a means to settle disputes, but this may be a mistaken policy. Men, and women as well, would benefit from having a forum to physically confront their opponents—say, an organized sports competition in which serious physical injury could be avoided—after they have fully aired their points of view in verbal discourse. This is an ancient vertebrate heritage. Here, finally, is a constructive use of the sport of boxing, using adequately padded gloves and sufficient head protection. Advantages accruing to society would be tremendous. A socially condoned outlet for non-destructive violence aimed at the source of frustration would prevent many antisocial, intrafamilial, displaced violent acts now all too common. Not only would individuals have less stress-induced illness, but interpersonal animosities masquerading as true doctrinal, scientific, and policy differences would be significantly diminished.

Aggression and stress can also be significantly reduced by vicariously experiencing contests and sports events. Small-scale warfare has been a part of human history as far back as records extend, and it is very likely that intergroup conflict goes back to primate origins. Sports are a harmless surrogate for small-scale warfare and have beneficial effects for both participants and observers. As Nobelist Konrad Lorenz noted in his 1992 book *On Aggression*, vicariously experiencing a meaningful contest can be a remarkably effective antidote to interpersonal aggression on a large scale.

Above and beyond causes of stress from interpersonal and societal causes, the environment in which you live can be very stressful. As discussed in chapter 13, environments made marginal by air or water pollution, excessive noise, crowding, deforestation, poor shelter, or just plain ugly surroundings can be a prison. From a comparative primatological standpoint, humans in such environments are comparable to monkeys crowded into zoo cages, subject to disease, both physical and emotional. The evolutionary solutions are to improve your environment, or to escape to a more optimal environment. Biologist E. O. Wilson suggests that there is a fundamental "biophilia" in humans, born of millions of years of coevolution and living with other species of plants and animals, that must be satisfied if we are to be happy and well-adjusted in our environment.[38] A similar theme is sounded by anthropologist Lionel Tiger in *The Pursuit of Pleasure*,[39] where he maintains that there is an evolutionary right of all humans to water, light, trees, fresh air, and open spaces in their living environments. Many physicians may think that such environmental stressors are not medical problems, but from evolutionary and preventive perspectives, they are. They are also, of course, economic, sociological, and political problems, leading us to agree again with E. O. Wilson when he suggests that "consilience"—a meeting of minds from disparate disciplines with a common enlightened agenda—is far overdue.[40]

Evolving Back to Health in the United States

In 1911, anthropologist Franz Boas discovered that the children of immigrants to the United States were taller, heavier, more robust, and even had different skull shapes than their parents.[41] The implications were far-reaching. Not only was it clear that environment plays a very important role in peoples' physical attributes, thus mitigating the immutability of race and biological inheritance, but an unmistakable subtheme was that the United States was a healthy place in which to grow up. In contrast, nearly a hundred years later, a number of studies[42] have demonstrated a surprising "healthy migrant" phenomenon—immigrants to the United States and other Western nations are now much less prone to develop chronic long-term disease than are native-born and -bred Americans. Apparently, the unhealthy aspects of modern American and Western lifestyles have caught up with us, and they now exceed the capabilities of our advanced medical facilities, public health systems, and nutritional potentialities, of which Western nations have been so proud. This is an unmistakable wake-up call to change lifestyles, diets, and social environments in the United States and other places like it. Because medical problems become exacerbated as we age, old age has now become a dreaded time of chronic disease, despondency, and depression. It need not be so.

Biological anthropologists look at old age in the human species as only the last stage of growth and development—that period of life in which the rate of cellular death begins to outpace the rate of cellular replication. This period of our lives is not merely a time when our bodies have worn out or when damage to cells and DNA have rendered bodily operations feeble. It is programmed. In analogy with apoptosis, or programmed cell death, the Russian gerontologist V. P. Skulachev has called this period of programmed organismal death "phenoptosis."[43] Some species, like salmon that lay eggs and then immediately die, undergo acute phenoptosis. Others, such as humans, undergo extended phenoptosis. We will eventually die, but there is no reason that we have to suffer tremendous morbidity before we get there.

We can explain a long postreproductive period in humans from the standpoint of its evolutionary advantages. Recalling our discussion of postreproductive life in primate social groups in the context of the evolution of menopause, it is clear that the social benefits accruing to the group, and the inclusive fitness conferred on such individuals by natural selection, account for this phenomenon. But this postreproductive old age has become a major focus of modern medicine because it is a time fraught with illness, mental disorders, and debilitating disease. Most of the billions of dollars spent in health care each year are spent on treatment and hospitalization for the aged. For many of us, old age and disease go hand in hand, and are virtually synonymous. Is there any other way to think of them?

Yes. In hunter-gatherer societies around the world, old people do not gain weight as they age. Starting out as fit, physically strong adults, they maintain good muscle mass, strength, and low fat-to-muscle ratios into advanced age. They do not suffer from diabetes, high blood pressure, heart attack, stroke, osteoporosis, inflammatory bowel disease, cancers, or the myriad of other standard ailments that affect aged Westerners. Older men and women take part in daily life along with their children, grandchildren, relatives, and friends, although usually in less physically demanding roles. Two intertwined aspects of human biology seem essential for maintaining vitality into old age—staying lean and strong (whether you are male or female), and staying active, the "use-it-or-lose-it" principle. If you can maintain these two aspects of your body, modern medicine can help you overcome the odd pathogenic organism, wear-and-tear problems such as osteoarthritis, or even rather major injuries, any of which could have done in our hunter-gatherer ancestors. You do have some advantages living in the 21st century.

If we follow the guidelines of evolutionary medicine and live well into advanced age, what is our maximum life span? Theoretical estimates based on both fossil hominid samples[44] and comparative studies of living primates suggest that human beings can live to about 120 years old. Living to this age is hard to imagine for most of us. Would we want to survive that long, even if we could?

To answer that question, I went to visit the oldest living person in the world. She is a delightful lady known by the nickname of "Ma Pampo," who lives on the Caribbean island of Dominica. Her real name is Elizabeth Isreal, and church records show that she was born on January 27, 1875, making her 126 years old when I met her, in 2001. (Queen Victoria was on the English throne and Ulysses S. Grant was president of the United States when she was born). Today, still wiry and muscular at 90 pounds, Ma Pampo is alert, listens to the radio, visits with friends and relatives, and still votes in Dominican elections. She worked for 90 years on a lime and cocoa plantation, retiring at age 104. The work was hard—carrying heavy sacks of limes from the trees, and "coco-dancing" on the cacao beans to dehusk them. Still endowed with a strong grip, she has been healthy her entire life. She recently received Britain's Princess Anne and gave her some basil and bay leaf from her garden to make tea for her grandmother, the Queen Mother, "so that she could live longer." She is surrounded by friends and family. The keys to Ma Pampo's long life are her activity, cardiovascular fitness, leanness, and muscular strength. She has had a good life, and she still does. Looking at Ma Pampo's now wrinkled visage, you could think of her as a face out of the past, but I prefer to believe that she presages our future—a future that holds out health and longevity as gifts from our evolutionary past.

The Evolution of Senescence and Death

There are two evolutionary schools of thought regarding senescence and death. One is the "antagonistic pleiotropy" school, which maintains that natural selection concentrates its action on the young, reproductively active period of life. Characteristics that maximize reproductive success up to and including this stage of life are favored; characteristics of old age are just left over ("pleiotropic") and largely invisible to natural selection. This view of senescence is championed by George Williams.[45]

The other point of view is phenoptosis—that the age of death within a species is programmed by evolution, analogous to the programmed cell death now generally accepted to occur in normal growth and development and known as apoptosis. The early geneticist August Weismann argued that individuals in populations had to die, if evolution was to take place, so that progeny would have room to survive and reproduce. The variability in life spans across species (for example, the long life of a tortoise versus the short life of a hummingbird) makes most sense from a standpoint of natural selection, and there is increasing evidence that genes control longevity.[46]

The two perspectives hold more than academic interest, because each point of view implies a different treatment for old-age ailments, common medical problems in senescence, and prevention. For example, Drs. Joseph Raffaele and Ronald Livesey are internal medicine physicians with a clinic specializing in antiaging medicine in New York City.[47] The antagonistic pleiotropy theory underlies their treatment regime, which involves sex and growth hormonal replacement therapy to levels characteristic of a 25-year-old. There are, of course, many more hormones in the body and a bewildering endocrinological complexity that is still being discovered. Modifying some but not others may have unintended but significant side effects. For the moment, I'll bet on Ma Pampo's approach.

Web-based Resources on Evolutionary Human Diets

Beyond Vegetarianism
www.beyondveg.com/index.shtml

Iowa State University's Tasty Insect Recipes
www.ent.iastate.edu/misc/insectsasfood.html

NeanderTim—a Caveman's Guide to Nutrition
www.sofdesign.com/neander

Paleofood Links
www.plab.ku.dk/tcbh/paleofood-links.htm

The Paleolithic Diet Page: What the Hunter/Gatherers Ate
www.panix.com/~paleodiet

University of Kentucky Entomology's Bugfood III: Insect Snacks from around the World
www.uky.edu/Agriculture/Entomology/ythfacts/bugfood/yf8 13.htm

What Is the Healthiest Diet for the Human Animal?
www.naturalhub.com/opinion_right_food_for_the_human_ animal.htm

Notes

Introduction

1. Oliwenstein, Lori. 1995. Dr. Darwin. Discover Magazine 19:111–117.

Chapter 1. Achieving Adaptive Normality, Your Evolutionary Birthright

1. McFarland, D. 1999. Animal Behaviour: Psychobiology, Ethology, and Evolution. Harlow, U.K.: Longman.
2. Little, M.A., and R. Garruto. 2000. Human adaptability research into the beginning of the third millennium. Hum. Biol. 72:179–199; Kurland, J.A. 1985. Optimal foraging strategy and hominid evolution: Labor and reciprocity. Amer. Anthropologist 87:73–93; Orians, G.H., and J.H. Heerwagen. 1992. Evolved responses to landscapes. In: Barkow, J.H. et al., eds. The Adapted Min
. New York: Cambridge University Press.
3. Ciochon, R., and R. Larick. 1996. The African Emergence and Early Asian Dispersals of the Genus *Homo*. American Scientist 84(6):538–551.
4. Boaz, Noel T. 1997. Eco Homo. New York: Basic.
5. Boaz, N.T. 1979. Early hominid population densities: New estimates. Science 206:592–595.
6. A pseudonym, like other individual patient names mentioned in this book.
7. Burkitt, D.P. 1973. Some diseases characteristic of modern western civilization: A possible common causative factor. Clin. Radiol. 24:271–280; Nesse, R.M. 2001. How is Darwinian medicine useful? Western J. Med. 174:358–360.; Konner, M. 2001. Evolution and our environment: Will we adapt? Western J. Med. 174:360–361.

Chapter 2. How Our Health Evolved

1. Mayr, Ernst. 1991. One Long Argument: Charles Darwin and the Genesis of Modern Evolutionary Thought. Cambridge, Mass.: Harvard University Press.
2. Gesteland, Raymond F., Thomas R. Cech, and John F. Atkins, eds. 1999. The RNA World, 2nd ed. Cold Spring Harbor Monograph Series 37. Cold Spring Harbor, N.Y.: Cold Spring Harbor Press.
3. Morowitz, H.J., et al. 2000. The origin of intermediary metabolism. Proc. Nat. Acad. Sci. 97:7704–7708.

4. Sverdlov, E.D. 2000. Retroviruses and primate evolution. BioEssays 22:161–171.; Travis, J. 2000. Do captured viral genes make human pregnancies possible? Science News, May 13, 2000.

5. Margulis, L, and D. Sagan. 1986. Microcosmos: Four Billion Years of Evolution from Our Microbial Ancestors. New York: Summit.

6. Wang, D. Y.-C., S. Kumar, and S. B. Hedges. 1999. Divergence time estimates for the early history of animal phyla and the origin of plants, animals, and fungi. Proc. Roy. Soc. London B 266:163–171.

7. Michod, R.E., and D. Roze. 2001. Cooperation and conflict in the evolution of multicellularity. Heredity 86:1–7.

8. Wainwright, P.O., et al. 1993. Monophyletic origins of the metazoa: An evolutionary link with fungi. Science 260:340–342.

9. The three germ layers of the embryo are termed the "ectoderm," which gives rise to most of the brain, eyes, nerves, skin, and other scattered structures near the outside of the body; the "mesoderm," which gives rise to muscle, heart and circulatory system, blood, and many components of internal organs; and the "endoderm," which gives rise to most structures of the digestive system.

10. Briggs, Derke E.G., Douglas H. Erwin, and Frederick J. Collier. 1994. The Fossils of the Burgess Shale. Washington, D.C.: Smithsonian Institution Press.

11. A term referring a broad array of early and poorly known early primates, from the genus name *Plesiadapis,* and dating from the Paleocene and Eocene epochs (65 to 40 million years ago).

12. Cartmill, M. 1974. Rethinking primate origins. Science 184:436–443.

13. Pollock, J.I., and R.J. Mullin. 1987. Vitamin C biosynthesis in prosimians: Evidence for the anthropoid affinity of Tarsius. Amer. J. Phys. Anthrop. 73:65–70; Banhegyi, G., et al. 1997. Ascorbate metabolism and its regulation in animals. Free Rad. Biol. Med. 23:793–803.

14. Simons, E.L. 1990. Discovery of the oldest known anthropoidean skull from the Paleogene of Egypt. Science 247:1567–1569.

15. Darwin, C.R. 1872. Descent of Man. London: Murray.

16. Boaz, Noel T. 1997. Eco Homo. New York: Basic.

17. Trevathan W. 1999. Evolutionary obstetrics. In: Trevathan, W.R., E.O. Smith, and J.J. McKenna, eds. Evolutionary Medicine, pp. 183–207. New York: Oxford University Press.

18. Armelagos, G.J., K.C. Barnes, and J. Lin. 1998. Disease in human evolution. In: Selig, R.O., and M.R. London, eds. Anthropology Explored, pp. 96–105. Washington, D.C: Smithsonian Institution Press.

19. Ewald, P.W. 1994. Evolution of Infectious Disease. New York: Oxford University Press.

Chapter 3. An Evolutionary Child's Birthright: Perinatal and Pediatric Diseases

1. Haeckel, Ernst. 1868. Naturliche Schopfungsgeschichte. Berlin: Reimer.

2. The allusion to seal flippers, adaptations in these aquatic vertebrates evolved from their land-living, four-footed ancestors, is inaccurate insofar as the flipper- or paddlelike limbs of thalidomide children simply never developed. They are more accurately to be compared with the fins of primitive fish, such as the living lobe-fin fish, the coelacanth. The term "meromelia," meaning "partial limbs," is a preferable term for the birth defect.

3. Named after Dr. J.L. H Down, an English pediatrician who named the condition in 1866.

4. "Placenta" is the Latin word for a flat cake, whose appearance suggests a similarity in form to the human organ.

5. The pharmaceutical companies distanced themselves as far as possible from thalidomide for years because of potential association with human birth defects. Only in the last five years, with approval of the U.S. Food and Drug Administration (FDA) of thalidomide for use in cancer and AIDS treatment, has research on its mechanism of action resumed.

6. Profet, M. 1991. The function of allergy: Immunological defense against toxins. Quart. Rev. Biol. 66:23–62.

7. Flaxman S.M., and P.W. Sherman. 2000. Morning sickness: A mechanism for protecting mother and embryo. Quart. Rev. Biol. 75(2):113–148.

8. Martin, Robert. 1980. James Arthur Lecture of the Evolution of the Human Brain. New York: American Museum of Natural History.

9. Trevathan, Wenda. 1996. The evolution of bipedalism and assisted birth. Med. Anthropol. Quart. 10(2):287–290; Idem. 1999. Evolutionary obstetrics. In: Trevathan, W.R., E.O. Smith, and J.J. McKenna, eds. Evolutionary Medicine, pp. 183–207. New York: Oxford University Press.

10. "Cyanosis" literally means "blue," but this appellation only accurately refers to light-skinned babies. Dark-skinned cyanotic babies tend to be grayish in color, but the lack of oxygenation of tissues from a heart defect is just as acute.

11. Brett, John, and S. Niermeyer. 1999. Is neonatal jaundice a disease or an adaptive process? In: Trevathan, W.R., E.O. Smith, and J.J. McKenna, eds. Evolutionary Medicine, pp. 7–25. New York: Oxford University Press.

12. McKenna, J.J., S. Mosko, and C. Richard. 1999. Breastfeeding and mother-infant cosleeping in relation to SIDS prevention. In: Trevathan, W.R., E.O. Smith, and J.J. McKenna, eds. Evolutionary Medicine, pp. 53–74. New York: Oxford University Press.

13. Profet, M. 1991. The function of allergy: Immunological defense against toxins. Quart. Rev. Biol. 66:23–62, Barnes, K.C., G.J. Armelagos, and S.C. Morreale. 1999. Darwinian medicine and the emergence of allergy. In: Trevathan, W.R., E.O. Smith, and J.J. McKenna, eds. Evolutionary Medicine, pp. 209–243. New York: Oxford University Press.

14. Aveskogh, M., and L. Hellman. 1998. Evidence for an early appearance of modern post-switch isotypes in mammalian evolution; cloning of IgE, IgG and IgA from the marsupial *Monodelphis domestica*. Eur. J. Immunol. 9:2738–2750.

15. Fireman, P. 1997. Otitis media and eustachian tube dysfunction: Connection to allergic rhinitis. J. Allergy Clin. Immunol. 99(2):S787–S797.

16. Klein, J.O. 1994 Otitis media. Clin. Infect. Dis. 19(5):823–833.

17. Shu, X.O. 1997. Epidemiology of childhood leukemia. Curr. Opin. Hematol. 4(4):227–232.

Chapter 4. The Virus War

1. Gesteland, Raymond F., Thomas R. Cech, and John F. Atkins, eds. 1999. The RNA World, 2nd ed. Cold Spring Harbor Monograph Series 37. Cold Spring Harbor, N.Y.: Cold Spring Harbor Press.

2. Flint, S.J., et al. 2000. Principles of Virology: Molecular Biology, Pathogenesis, and Control, pp. 696–701. Washington, D.C.: ASM Press.

3. Murphy, F.A. 1999. The evolution of viruses, the emergence of viral diseases: A synthesis that Martinus Beijerinck might enjoy. Arch. Virol. Suppl. 15:73–85.

4. Ewald, Paul W. 1994. Evolution of Infectious Disease. New York: Oxford University Press.

5. Love, J. 1998. "Chicken flu"—recombinant genes on the loose! Science Explained. Available at www.synapses.

6. Wendorf, M. 1999. Diabetes and enterovirus autoimmunity in glacial Europe. Med. Hypoth. 52:423–429.

Chapter 5. Cellular Stress: A General Model for Cancer

1. Benedek, T.G., and K.F. Kiple. 1993. Concepts of cancer. In: Kiple, K.F., ed., The Cambridge World History of Human Disease, pp. 102–110. Cambridge, U.K.: Cambridge University Press.

2. Braun, A.C. 1977. The Story of Cancer: On Its Nature, Causes, and Control. Reading, Mass.: Addison-Wesley.

3. Virchow, Rudolf. 1893. The place of pathology among the natural sciences. Trans. and repr. in: Rather, L.J., ed. 1958. Disease, Life, and Man: Selected Essays by Rudolf Virchow, pp. 151–169. Stanford, Calif.: Stanford University Press.

4. Virchow, Rudolf. 1877. Standpoints in scientific medicine. Trans. and repr. in: Rather, L.J., ed. 1958. Disease, Life, and Man: Selected Essays by Rudolf Virchow, pp. 142–150. Stanford, Calif.: Stanford University Press.

5. Simons, J. W. 2000. Coming of age: "Dysgenics"—a theory connecting induction of persistent delayed genomic instability with disturbed cellular ageing. Int. J. Radiat. Biol. 76(11):1533–1543.

6. Manson-Bahr, P. H. 1966. Manson's Tropical Diseases: A Manual of the Diseases of Warm Climates. London: Bailliére Tindall.

7. Benedek, T. G., and K. F. Kiple. 1993. Concepts of cancer. In: Kiple, K. F., ed. The Cambridge World History of Human Disease, p. 109. Cambridge, U.K.: Cambridge University Press.

8. Bhardwaj, S. M. 1993. Disease ecologies of South Asia. In: Kiple, K. F., ed., The Cambridge World History of Human Disease, pp. 463–476. Cambridge, U.K.: Cambridge University Press.

9. Rock, C. L. 1999. Diet therapy for cancer prevention. In: Harrison's Internal Medicine Online, chap. 77. Available at www.harisonson online.com.

Chapter 6. Breast Cancer, Prostate Diseases, and Cancers of the Reproductive System

1. Campbell, R. M., and C. G. Scances. 1992. Evolution of the growth hormone-releasing factor (GRF) family of peptides. Growth Regul. 2:175–191.

2. Sandor, T., and A. Z. Mehdi. 1979. Steroids and evolution. In: Barrington, E. J. W., ed. Hormones and Evolution, pp. 1–72. New York: Academic.

3. Bolander, F. F. 1994. Molecular Endocrinology, pp. 493–517. San Diego: Academic.

4. Murray, R. K., et al., eds. 2000. Harper's Biochemistry, 25th ed., p. 601. Stamford, Conn.: Appleton and Lange.

5. Eaton, S. B., et al. 1994. Women's reproductive cancers in evolutionary context. Quart. Rev. Biol. 69:353–367; Eaton, S. B., and S. B. Eaton III. 1999. Breast cancer in evolutionary context. In: Trevathan W. R., E. O. Smith, and J. J. McKenna, eds. Evolutionary Medicine, pp. 429–442. New York: Oxford University Press.

6. World Health Organization. 1998. About obesity. International obesity Task Force. Available at www.iaso.org/.

7. Rink, J. D., et al. 1996. Cellular characterization of adipose tissue from various body sites of women. J. Clin. Endocrinol. 81(7):2443–2447; Rubin, G. L., et al. 2000. Peroxisome proliferator-activated receptor gamma ligands inhibit estrogen biosynthesis in human breast adipose tissue: Possible implications for breast cancer. Cancer Res. 60(6):1604–1608.

8. Ries, L. A. G., et al. 2000. The annual report to the nation on the status of cancer, 1973–1997, with a special section on colorectal cancer. Cancer 88(10):2398–2424.

9. Murray, R.K., et al., eds. 2000. Harper's Biochemistry, 25th ed., p. 599. Stamford, Conn.: Appleton and Lange.

10. Sciarra, F., and V. Toscano. 2000. Role of estrogens in human benign prostatic hyperplasia. Arch. Androl. 44(3):213–220.

11. Jeyaraj, D.A., et al. 2000. Effects of long-term administration of androgens and estrogen on rhesus monkey prostate: Possible induction of benign prostatic hyperplasia. J. Androl. 21(6):833–841.

Chapter 7. Heart Disease and High Blood Pressure: A Story of Fish and Chips

1. Smith, H.W. 1961. From Fish to Philosopher. New York: American Museum of Natural History/Doubleday. This is an excellent natural history and evolutionary narrative of the evolution of the kidney.

2. Guyton, A.C. 1991. Textbook of Medical Physiology, 8th ed., pp. 209–211. Philadelphia: Saunders.

3. Tropea, B.I., et al. 2000. Reduction of aortic wall motion inhibits hypertension-mediated experimental atherosclerosis. Arteriosclr. Thromb. Vacs. Biol. 20(9):2127–2133.

4. Massie, B.M. 1997. Systemic hypertension. In: Tierney, L.M., et al., eds. Current Medical Diagnosis and Treatment, 36th ed., pp. 412–431. Stamford, Conn.: Appleton and Lange.

5. Howell, J.D. 1993. Concepts of heart-related diseases. In: Kiple, K.F., ed. The Cambridge World History of Human Disease, pp. 91–102. Cambridge, U.K.: Cambridge University Press.

6. Wilson, T.W., and C.E. Grim. 1993. Hypertension. In: Kiple, K.F., ed. The Cambridge World History of Human Disease, pp. 789–794. Cambridge, U.K.: Cambridge University Press.

7. Lindeberg, S., et al. 1994. Cardiovascular risk factors in a Melanesian population apparently free from stroke and ischaemic heart disease—the Kitava study. J. Intern. Med. 236:331–334.

8. Smith, H.W. 1956. Kamongo; or, the Lungfish and the Padre. New York: Viking.

9. Olson, K.R., et al. 1987. Angiotensin-converting enzyme in organs of air-breathing fish. Gen. Comp. Endocrinol. 68(3):486–491.

10. Pauletto, P., et al. 1999. Factors underlying the increase in carotid intima-media thickness in borderline hypertensives. Arteriosclr. Thromb. Vasc. Biol. 19(5):1231–1237.

11. Wilson, T.W. 1986. Africa, Afro-Americans, and hypertension: An hypothesis. Social Sciences History 10:489–500.

12. De Wardener, H.E. 1996. Sodium and hypertension. Arch. Mal. Coeur Vaiss. 89, Spec. No. 4.

Chapter 8. Why We Smoke

1. Kalant, H., and W.H.E. Roschlau. 1998. Principles of Medical Pharmacology, 6th ed., pp. 156–157. New York: Oxford University Press.

2. Jones, S., S. Sudweeks, and J.L. Yakel. 1999. Nicotinic receptors in the brain. Trends Neurosci. 22(12):555–561; Melichar, J.K., et al. 2001. Addiction and withdrawal—current views. Curr. Opinion Pharm. 1(1):84–90.

3. Ernster, V.L., et al. 1994. Epidemiology of lung cancer. In: Murray, J.F., and J.A. Nadel, eds. Textbook of Respiratory Medicine, vol. 2, pp. 1504–1527. Philadelphia: Saunders.

4. Chia, M.M., et al. 1994. Biology of lung cancer. In: Murray, J.F., and J.A. Nadel, eds. Textbook of Respiratory Medicine, vol. 2, pp. 1485–1503. Philadelphia: Saunders.

5. Cantor, J.O., and G.M. Turino. 1991. Animal models of emphysema. In: Cherniak, N.S., ed. Chronic Obstructive Pulmonary Disease, pp. 63–69. Philadelphia: Saunders.

6. DeNelsky, G.Y., and T.L. Plesec. 1993. Smoking and smoking cessation. In: Matzen, R.N., and R.S. Lang, eds. Clinical Preventive Medicine, pp. 256–281. St. Louis: Mosby.

7. Rioux, N., and A. Castouquay. 2000. The induction of cyclooxygenase-1 by a tobacco carcinogen in U937 human macrophages is correlated to the activation of NF-kappaB. Carcinogenesis 2(9):1745–1751.

8. Lang, R.S. 1993. Lung cancer. In: Matzen, R.N., and R.S. Lang, eds. Clinical Preventive Medicine, p. 917–927. St. Louis: Mosby.

Chapter 9. Diabetes Mellitus and the "Thrifty Genotype"

1. There are several types of diabetes, the main ones being type I, in which children are primarily affected and the insulin-secreting (beta) cells of the pancreas are destroyed, and type II, diabetes mellitus, in which the beta cells produce insulin that the body's cells cannot use. Diabetes insipidus is a rare third form in which the pituitary gland fails to produce antidiuretic hormone (ADH).

2. Neel, J.V. 1962. Diabetes mellitus: A "thrifty genotype" rendered detrimental by "progress." Amer. J. Hum. Genet. 14:353–362.

3. An old anatomical mnemonic tells us that "the pancreas lies in the arms of the duodenum [on the right side below the stomach] and tickles the spleen with her feet [on the left side deep to the rib cage]."

4. Insulin gets its name from the fact it comes from little "insulas," or islets of cells, known as the islets of Langerhans within the pancreas.

5. Glycosuria is the "spilling," or excretion of glucose, into the urine when the amount in the bloodstream is in excess of the kidney tubules' ability to reabsorb it.

6. Glucagon binds to a G ("guanine-nucleotide-binding")-protein-linked receptor molecule, while insulin binds to an enzyme-linked (tyrosine kinase) receptor.

7. Felig P., et al. 1976. Insulin, glucagon, and somatostatin in normal physiology and diabetes mellitus. Diabetes 12:1091–1099.

8. Tokuyama, Y., et al. 1995. Evolution of beta-cell dysfunction in the male Zucker diabetic fatty rat. Diabetes 12:1447–1457.

9. Donath, M.Y., et al. 1999. Hyperglycemia-induced beta-cell apoptosis in pancreatic islets of *Psammomys obesus* during development of diabetes. Diabetes 48(4):738–744.

10. Bailey, C.J. 2000. Potential new treatments for type 2 diabetes. Trends Pharm. Sci. 21(7):259–265.

Chapter 10. Gout, Liver Enzymes, and Global Climate Change

1. Orowan, E. 1955. The origin of man. Nature 175:683–684.

2. Ames, B.N., et al. 1981. Uric acid provides an antioxidant defense in humans against oxidant- and radical-caused aging and cancer: A hypothesis. Proc. Natl. Acad. Sci. 78(11):6858–6862.

3. Despite a long-held and widely cited belief that the Dalmatian dog lacked the enzyme urate oxidase, in fact, research dating back to 1938, published by H.C. Trimble and C.E. Keeler in the *Journal of Heredity* (vol. 29, p. 280), showed that the enzyme is present and functional in this breed of dog, but that the presence of uric acid in its urine was due to a failure of the kidney tubules to reabsorb uric acid. This type of uricosuria in the Dalmatian is genetically inherited as a recessive trait. The net effect of the kidneys' failure to reabsorb uric acid, however, would serve to conserve water because more (insoluble) uric acid would be excreted and more water would be reabsorbed by the kidney's tubules.

4. Wynn, J.G., and G.J. Retallack. 2001. Paleoenvironmental reconstruction of middle Miocene paleosols bearing *Kenyapithecus* and *Victoriapithecus*, Nyakach Formation, southwestern Kenya. J. Hum. Evol. 40:263–288.

5. Ward, S., et al. 1999. *Equatorius:* A new hominoid genus from the middle Miocene of Kenya. Science 285:1382–1386.

6. Scott, R.S., J. Kappelman, and J. Kelley. 1999. The paleoenvironment of *Sivapithecus parvada*. J. Hum. Evol. 36:245–274.

7. Boaz, N.T. 1994. Significance of the Western Rift for hominid origins. In: R.S. Corruccini and R.L. Ciochon, eds. Integrative Paths to the Past: Paleoanthropological Advances in Honor of F.C. Howell, pp. 321–343. New York: Prentice-Hall.

8. Wu, X., et al. 1992. Two independent mutational events in the loss of urate oxidase during hominoid evolution. J. Mol. Evol. 34:78–84.

9. Hypoxanthine-guanine phosphoribosyltransferase, the most important of the enzymes involved in the so-called salvage purine pathway, normally adds a phosphate to the purines hypoxanthine and guanine to form nucleotides, important in DNA and RNA in the body.

Chapter 11. Back Pain, Bad Knees, and Flatfeet

1. Putz, R.L., and M. Muller-Gerbl. 1996. The vertebral column—a phylogenetic failure? A theory explaining the function and vulnerability of the human spine. Clin. Anat. 9:205–212.

2. Shapiro, L.J., and W.L. Jungers. 1988. Back muscle function during bipedal walking in chimpanzee and gibbon: Implications for the evolution of human locomotion. Amer. J. Phys. Anthrop. 77:201–212.

3. Kidd, R. 1999. Evolution of the rearfoot: A model of adaptation with evidence from the fossil record. J. Amer. Med. Assoc. 89:2–17.

4. Tetley, Michael. 2000. Instinctive sleeping and resting postures: An anthropological and zoological approach to treatment of low back and joint pain. Brit. Med. J. 321:1616–1618.

5. Olson, T.R., and M.R. Seidel. 1983. The evolutionary basis of some clinical disorders of the human foot: A comparative survey of the primates. Foot and Ankle 3:322–341; Moorehead, J., and L. Wobeskya. 1995. Evolutionary aspects of foot disorders. J. Amer. Podiatr. Med. Assoc. 85:209–213.

6. Lee, R.B. and I. Devore, eds. 1968. Man the Hunter. Chicago: Aldine; Barnard, A. 1992. Hunters and Herders of Southern Africa: A Comparative Ethnography of the Khoisan Peoples. Cambridge, U.K.: Cambridge University Press.

7. Sheon, R.P. 1997. Repetitive strain injury: 2. Diagnostic and treatment tips on six common problems. Goff Group. Postgrad. Med. 102:72–78; Nainzedeh, N., et al. 1999. Repetitive strain injury (cumulative trauma disorder): Causes and treatment. Mt. Sinai J. Med. 66:192–196.

8. Russell, I.J. 1999. Is fibromyalgia a distinct clinical entity? The clinical investigator's evidence. Baillieres Best Pract. Res. Clin. Rheumatol. 13:445–454.

Chapter 12. Gut Diseases

1. Atkins, R.C. 1992. Dr. Atkins' New Diet Revolution. New York: Avon Books.

2. USDA. 1995. Nutrition and Your Health: Dietary Guidelines for Americans, 4th ed. Washington, D.C.: U.S. Government Printing Office.

3. Somer, Elizabeth. 2001. The Origin Diet: How Eating in Tune with Your Evolutionary Roots Can Prevent Disease, Boost Vitality and Help You Stay Lean and Fit. New York: Henry Holt.

4. Pauling, L. 1986. How to Live Longer and Feel Better. New York: W.H. Freeman.

5. Peters, C. 1981. Robust versus gracile early hominid masticatory capabilities: The advantages of the megadonts. Anthrop. UCLA 7(1–2):161–181.

6. Popovich, D.G., et al. 1997. The western lowland gorilla diet has implications for the health of humans and other hominoids. J. Nutr. 127:2000–2005.

7. Aiello, L.C., and P. Wheeler. 1995. The expensive tissue hypothesis: The brain and the digestive system in human and primate evolution. Curr. Anthrop. 36:199–221.

8. Fiber is indigestible material in food that stimulates the wavelike muscular actions of the intestinal walls known as "peristalsis."

9. Semaw, S., et al. 1997. 2.5-million-year-old stone tools from Gona, Ethiopia. Nature 385:333–336.

10. Flannery, T. 2001. The Eternal Frontier: An Ecological History of North America and Its Peoples. New York: Atlantic Monthly.

11. Eaton, S.B., S.B. Eaton III, and M.J. Konner. 1999. Paleolithic nutrition revisited. In: Trevathan W.R., E.O. Smith, and J.J. McKenna, eds. Evolutionary Medicine, pp. 313–332. New York: Oxford University Press.

12. Eaton, S.B., M. Shostak, and M. Konner. 1988. The Paleolithic Prescription: A Program of Diet and Exercise and a Design for Living. pp. 92–93. New York: Harper and Row.

13. Fauci, A.S., et al., eds. 1998. Harrison's Principles of Internal Medicine, 14th ed., p. 1646. New York: McGraw-Hill.

14. Boaz, N.T., and F.C. Howell. 1977. A gracile hominid cranium from upper Member G of the Shungura Formation, Ethiopia. Amer. J. Phys. Anthrop. 46:93–108.

15. Marshall, B.J. 1995 Helicobacter pylori in peptic ulcer: Have Koch's postulates been fulfilled? Ann. Med. 27:565–568.

16. Wood, J.D., et al. 1998. Colitis and colon cancer in cotton-top tamarins (Saguinus oedipus oedipus) living wild in their natural habitat. Dig. Dis. Sci. 43:1443–1453.

17. Boyle, P., and J.S. Langman. 2000. Clinical review: ABC of colorectal cancer. Brit. Med. J. 321:805–808.

18. Although our skin is the largest organ in the body, its epidermis is impervious to most microorganisms and chemicals, and, unlike the gastrointestinal tract, it is not functionally designed for absorption of environmental compounds.

19. Chambers, S., L. Evans, and A. Krishnan. 2001. Colorectal cancer among users of aspirin and nonsteroidal anti-inflammatory drugs. Epidemiol. 12:471–472; Terry, P., et al. 2001. Coffee consumption and risk of colorectal cancer in a population-based prospective cohort of Swedish women. Gut 49:87–90.

Chapter 13. *The Evolution of Psychiatric Disorders*

1. Darwin, C.R. 1872. The Expression of the Emotions in Man and Animals. London: Murray.

2. McGuire, M.T., and A. Troisi. 1998. Darwinian Psychiatry. New York: Oxford University Press.

3. Morris, D. 1969. The Human Zoo. London: Cape.

4. Zuckerman, S. 1932. The Social Life of Monkeys and Apes. New York: Harcourt Brace.

5. Harrison, P.J., D.L. Macmillan, and H.M. Young. 1995. Serotonin immunoreactivity in the ventral nerve cord of the primitive crustacean *Anaspides tasmaniae* closely resembles that of crayfish. J. Exp. Biol. 198:531–535.

6. MacLean, P. 1990. The Triune Brain in Evolution: Role in Paleocerebral Functions. New York: Plenum.

7. A part of the lower forebrain important in regulating autonomic bodily functions, such as food intake; sometimes considered the "head ganglion," or bundle of nerve cells of the sympathic nervous system, which mediates our fight-or-flight responses; literally "below the thalamus."

8. A part of the lower temporal lobe of the cerebrum, important in memory functions, thought by some 19th-century anatomists to separate the human brain from the ape brain; disproved by T.H. Huxley.

9. An almond-shaped nucleus of cells in the temporal lobe shown by physiological experiments to be important in emotions in mammals.

10. Gershon, M. 2000. The Second Brain: The Scientific Basis of Gut Instinct and a Groundbreaking New Understanding of Nervous Disorders of the Stomach and Intestines. New York: HarperCollins.

11. Shelley-Tremblay, J.F., and L.A. Rosén. 1996. Attention deficit hyperactivity disorder: An evolutionary perspective. J. Genet. Psychol. 157(4):443–453.

12. Baird, J., J.C. Stevenson, and D.C. Williams. 2000. The evolution of ADHD: A disorder of communication? Quart. Rev. Biol. 75(1):17–35.

13. Jerison, H.J. 1973. Evolution of the Brain and Intelligence. New York: Academic.

14. Crow, T.J. 1997. Is schizophrenia the price that Homo sapiens pays for language? Schizophr. Res. 28:127–141.

15. Jarvik, L.F., and B.S. Deckard. 1977. The Odyssean personality: A survival advantage for carriers of genes predisposing to schizophrenia? Neuropsychobiol. 3:179–191.

16. Bradshaw, J.L., and D.M. Sheppard. 2000. The neurodevelopmental frontostriatal disorders: Evolutionary adaptiveness and anomalous lateralization. Brain Lang. 73(2):297–320.

17. Four categories of endogenous opioids are now recognized: enkephalins (binding strongly to sigma receptors), endorphins (binding to mu and sigma receptors), dynorphins (binding to kappa and mu receptors), and endomorphins (binding strongly to mu receptors).

18. Dudley, R. 2000. Evolutionary origins of human alcoholism in primate frugivory. Quart. Rev. Biol. 75:3–15.

19. Blum K., et al. 2000. Reward deficiency syndrome: A biogenetic model for the diagnosis and treatment of impulsive, addictive, and compulsive behaviors. J. Psychoactive Drugs 32, Suppl.:i–iv, 1–112.

20. Nesse, Randolph M., and Kent C. Berridge. 1997. Psychoactive drug use in evolutionary perspective. Science 278:63–66.

Chapter 14. Uncivilized Solutions: Reestablishing Adaptive Normality in Your Life

1. Williams, G.C. 2000. The Raymond Pearl lecture, 1997: The quest for medical normalcy—who needs it? Amer. J. Hum. Biol. 12:10–16.

2. Eaton, S.B., S.B. Eaton III, and M.J. Konner. 1999. Paleolithic nutrition revisited. In: Trevathan, W.R., E.O. Smith, and J.J. McKenna, eds. Evolutionary Medicine, pp. 313–332. New York: Oxford University Press.

3. To obtain 3,000 calories per day, hunter-gatherers eat on average five pounds of food (Eaton, S.B., M. Shostak, and M. Konner. 1988. The Paleolithic Prescription: A Program of Diet and Exercise and a Design for Living, p. 63. New York: Harper and Row). The same caloric content in modern processed food is contained in 50 percent or less of modern supermarket food because of significantly less fiber and processing.

4. Available at www.pcrm.org/health/Info_on_Veg_Diets/vegetarian_foods.html.

5. Nestle, M. 2000. Paleolithic diets: A sceptical view. Nutr. Bull. 25(1):43–47.

6. Sponheimer, M., and J.A. Lee-Thorp. 1999. Isotopic evidence for the diet of an early hominid, Australopithecus africanus. Science 283:368–370.

7. Backwell, L.R., and F. d'Errico. 2001. Evidence of termite foraging by Swartkrans early hominids. Proc. Nat. Acad. Sci. 98:1358–1363.

8. Ames, B.N., M. Profet, and L.S. Gold. 1990. Dietary pesticides (99.99 percent all natural). Proc. Natl. Acad. Sci. 87:7777–7781.

9. Peterson, B. 1987. The Original Road Kill Cookbook. Berkeley, Calif.: Ten Speed Press.

10. Hubbard, K. 1998. Book review of The Eat a Bug Cookbook. Discover 19(8):97.

11. Gordon, David George. 1998. The Eat-a-Bug Cookbook: 33 Ways to Cook Grasshoppers, Ants, Water Bugs, Spiders, Centipedes and Their Kin. Berkeley, Calif.: Ten Speed Press.

12. Ramos-Elorduy, J. 1998. Creepy Crawly Cuisine: The Gourmet Guide to Edible Insects. Rochester, V.: Park Street Press.

13. Roosevelt, Theodore. 1910. African Game Trails: An Account of the African Wanderings of an American Hunter-Naturalist. New York: Scribner.

14. Eaton, S. B., M. Shostak, and M. Konner. 1988. The Paleolithic Prescription: A Program of Diet and Exercise and a Design for Living. New York: Harper and Row.

15. Dudley, R. 2000. Evolutionary origins of human alcoholism in primate frugivory. Quar. Rev. Biol. 75:3–15.

16. Smith, A. D., et al., eds. 1997. Oxford Dictionary of Biochemistry and Molecular Biology, p. 683. New York: Oxford University Press.

17. Maden, M. The effect of vitamin A (retinoids) on pattern formation implies a uniformity of developmental mechanisms throughout the animal kingdom. Acta Biother. 41:425–445.

18. Stryer, L. 1994. Biochemistry., pp. 452–453. New York: W. H. Freeman.

19. Doolittle, R. F. 1993. The evolution of vertebrate blood coagulation: A case of yin and yang. Thromb. Hem. 70:24–28.

20. Life Enhancement. The Science Behind the Products. 2001. Available at www.life-enhancement.com.

21. Gerber, L. M., G. C. Williams, and S. J. Gray. 1999. The nutrient-toxin dosage continuum in human evolution and health. Quart. Rev. Biol. 74:273–289.

22. Pauling, L. 1986. How to Live Longer and Feel Better. New York: W. H. Freeman.

23. Podmore, I. D., et al. 1998. Vitamin C exhibits pro-oxidant properties. Nature 392:550.

24. Morris, Paul J. 1993. The developmental role of the extracellular matrix suggests a monophyletic origin of the kingdom Animalia. Evolution 47:152–165.

25. Stone, I. 1972. The natural history of ascorbic acid in the evolution of mammals and primates and its significance for present day man. Orthomol. Psych. 1:82–89.

26. Banhegyi, G., et al. 1997. Ascorbate metabolism and its regulation in animals. Free Rad. Biol. Med. 23:793–803; Pollock, J. I., and R. J. Mullin. 1987. Vitamin C biosynthesis in prosimians: Evidence for the anthropoid affinity of Tarsius. Amer. J. Phys. Anthrop. 73:65–70.

27. Pall, M. 2000. Elevated, sustained peroxynitrite levels as the cause of chronic fatigue syndrome. Med. Hypo. 54:115–125.

28. Christen, S., et al. 1997. Gamma-tocopherol traps mutagenic electrophiles such as NO (X) and complements alpha-tocopherol: Physiolocical implications. Proc. Natl. Acad. Sci. 94:3217–3222.

29. National Institutes of Health, Clinical Nutrition Service. 2001. Facts about dietary supplements: Vitamin E. Available at www.cc.nih.gov/ccc/supplements.

30. Protor, P. H. 1989. Free radical and human disease. CRC Handbook Free Rad. Antiox. 1:209–221.

31. Neer, R. M. 1975. The evolutionary significance of vitamin D, skin pigment, and ultraviolet light. Amer. J. Phys. Anthrop. 43:409–416.

32. Jablonski, N. G., and G. Chaplin. 2000. The evolution of human skin coloration. J. Hum. Evol. 39:57–106.

33. Weinberg, E. D. 1984. Iron withholding: A defense against infection and neoplasia. Physiol. Rev. 64:65–102.

34. Centers for Disease Control, Atlanta, Georgia. Parasitic disease information: Hookworm infection. Available at www.cdc.gov/ncidod/dpd/para sites/hookworm.

35. Murray, P. R., et al. 1998. Medical Microbiology, 3rd ed. St. Louis: Mosby.

36. Marech, Rona. 1999. Mustn't see TV. Horizons, April 25, 1999. Available at www.thereporter.com/Current/Horizons/horiz042599.html.

37. "High Mileage Moms." Transact. Website of Surface Transportation Policy Project. Available at www.transact.org/Reports/highmilemoms/text.htm.

38. Wilson, E. O. 1984. Biophilia. Cambridge, Mass. Harvard University Press.

39. Tiger, Lionel. 1992. The Pursuit of Pleasure. New York: Little Brown.

40. Wilson, E. O. 1998. Consilience: The Unity of Knowledge. New York: Knopf.

41. Boas, Franz. 1911. Changes in Form of Body of Descendant of Immigrants. New York: n.p.

42. Razum, O., H. Zeeb, and S. Rohrman. 2000. The "healthy migrant effect"—not merely a fallacy of inaccurate denominator figures. Int. J. Epidemiol. 29:191–192; Che, J., E. Ng, and R. Wilkins. 1996. The health of Canada's immigrants in 1994–95. Health Rep. 7:33–45; Darmon, N., and M. Khlat. 2001. An overview of the health status of migrants in France, in relation to their dietary practices. Pub. Health Nutr. 4:163–172.

43. Skulachev, V. P. 1997. Aging is a specific biological function rather than the result of a disorder in complex living systems: Biochemical evidence in support of Weismann's hypothesis. Biochem. (Mosc.) 62:1191–1195.

44. Boaz, N. T. 1985. Early hominid paleoecology in the Omo basin, Ethiopia. In: Coppens, Y., ed. L'Environnement des Hominidés au Plio-Pléistocène, pp. 283–312. Paris: Fondation Singer-Polignac.

45. Williams, G. C. 1957. Pleiotropy, natural selection, and the evolution of senescence. Evolution 11:398–411.

46. Gems, D. Yeast longevity gene goes public. Nature 410:154–155.

47. Luddington, A. V. 2000. Antiaging medicine: Partners put evolutionary theory into practice. Geriatrics 55:37–46.

Index